Asthma therapy

D0224626

Peter J Barnes
Professor of Thoracic Medicine
Head of Respiratory Medicine
National Heart & Lung Institute
Imperial College
London

and

Simon Godfrey
Professor of Pediatrics
Director, Institute of Pulmonology
Hadassah University Hospital
Jerusalem
Israel

MARTIN DUNITZ

© Martin Dunitz 1998

First published in the United Kingdom in 1998 by

Martin Dunitz Ltd
The Livery House
7–9 Pratt Street
London NW1 0AE

A CIP record for this book is available from the British Library.

ISBN 1-85317-642-7

Distributed in the USA, Canada and Brazil
by

Blackwell Science Inc
Commerce Place
350 Main Street
Malden
MA 02148-5018
USA
Tel: 1-800-215-1000

Printed and bound in Italy by Printer Trento Srl.

Contents

Preface

Asthma has now become the commonest chronic
disease in industrialized countries and its prevalence
is increasing throughout the world. Asthma effects
all age groups and is often persistent so that 'there
is a lot of it about' and accounts for a large proportion of health care spending and loss of work. As a
result of an explosion of research in asthma with a
flood of scientific papers on every aspect of this
complex disease there have been major advances in
our understanding of its pathophysiology and this
has underpinned great improvements in its management over the last decade. In this short book we
have tried to summarize the rationale for current
therapy and to discuss the modern management of
asthma. This starts with an overview of the structural and functional changes in the disease, which
provides a basis for currently recommended treatments. We discuss the pharmacology of each drug
class now used in asthma therapy and how these
drugs are used in management. Guidelines for
asthma therapy have now been introduced in many

countries and we discuss the practical application of these guidelines in the day-to-day management of asthma. Some patients have particular problems that deserve special treatment and these issues are also discussed. Delivery devices for the inhalation of medications are as important as the drugs themselves and there have been important advances in these devices that make it much easier for the patient. Finally, we consider some of the new drugs now in development for asthma.

We hope that this book will provide a concise summary of modern asthma treatment and will be useful in the clinical management of this important disease.

Peter J Barnes, London
Simon Godfrey, Jerusalem

Pathophysiology of asthma

1

There have been important advances in our understanding of the pathophysiology of asthma and this
has led to a more rational approach to asthma
therapy. Asthma is a complex chronic inflammatory
disease that involves many inflammatory cells and
mediators, and in addition to bronchoconstriction
there are complex inflammatory effects on the
airways. In the past it was assumed that the basic
defect in asthma was abnormal contractility of
airway smooth muscle, giving rise to variable airflow
obstruction, and the common symptoms of intermittent wheeze and shortness of breath. However,
studies of airway smooth muscle from asthmatic
patients have shown no convincing evidence for
increased contractile responses to spasmogens such
as histamine in vitro, indicating that asthmatic
airway smooth muscle is not fundamentally abnormal and suggesting that it is the *control* of airway
calibre in vivo that is abnormal. For many years it
was assumed that mast cells played a critical role in
asthma and that mast cell mediators produce the

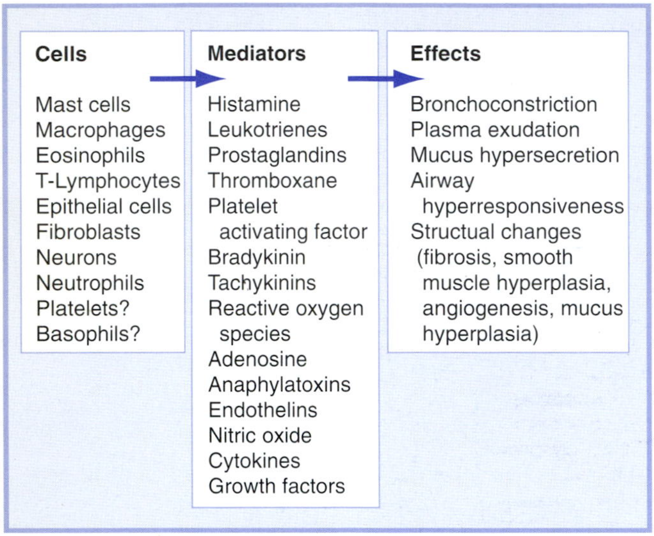

Cells	Mediators	Effects
Mast cells	Histamine	Bronchoconstriction
Macrophages	Leukotrienes	Plasma exudation
Eosinophils	Prostaglandins	Mucus hypersecretion
T-Lymphocytes	Thromboxane	Airway
Epithelial cells	Platelet	hyperresponsiveness
Fibroblasts	activating factor	Structual changes
Neurons	Bradykinin	(fibrosis, smooth
Neutrophils	Tachykinins	muscle hyperplasia,
Platelets?	Reactive oxygen	angiogenesis, mucus
Basophils?	species	hyperplasia)
	Adenosine	
	Anaphylatoxins	
	Endothelins	
	Nitric oxide	
	Cytokines	
	Growth factors	

Figure 1
Many cells, inflammatory mediators and inflammatory effects are involved in asthma

pathophysiology of asthma. More recently it has become clear that many different inflammatory cells are activated in asthmatic airways, and that these cells produce a variety of mediators that act in a complex manner on target cells of the airways to produce the abnormal pathophysiological features typical of asthma (**Figure 1**). Recent research has established that asthma, even in its mildest clinical forms, involves a special type of inflammation in the airways.

Asthma as an inflammatory disease

It has been recognized for many years that patients who die of asthma attacks have grossly inflamed airways. The airway wall is oedematous and infiltrated with inflammatory cells, which are predominantly eosinophils and lymphocytes. The airway epithelium is often shed in a patchy manner and clumps of epithelial cells are found in the airway lumen, which is often

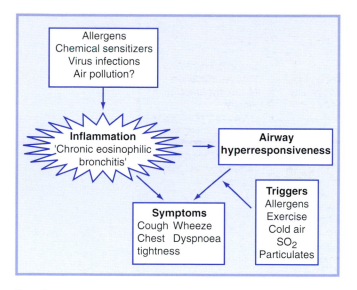

Figure 2
Inflammation in the airways of asthmatic patients leads to airway hyperresponsiveness and symptoms

occluded with a mucus plug. It is now clear that similar, although less intense, inflammatory changes are found in all asthmatic patients who are symptomatic. Even patients with episodic asthma have inflammatory changes at times when there are no symptoms. Fibreoptic bronchoscopy reveals that the airways of asthmatic patients are often reddened and swollen, indicating acute inflammation. Lavage has revealed an increase in the numbers of lymphocytes, mast cells and eosinophils and evidence for activation of macrophages in comparison with non-asthmatic controls. Biopsies have demonstrated increased numbers and activation of mast cells, macrophages, eosinophils and T-lymphocytes.

The relationship between inflammation and clinical symptoms of asthma is not clear. There is evidence that the degree of inflammation is related to airway hyperresponsiveness (AHR), as measured by inhaled histamine or

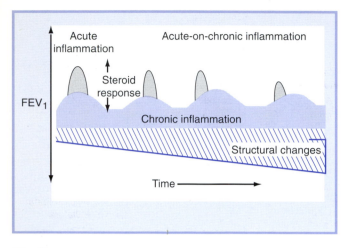

Figure 3
Asthma involves both acute and chronic inflammation. Continuing chronic inflammation may lead to structural changes that may underlie irreversible narrowing of the airways in asthma

methacholine challenge. Increased airway responsiveness is an exaggerated airway narrowing in response to many stimuli that is characteristic of asthma and the degree of AHR relates to asthma symptoms. Inflammation of the airways may increase airway responsiveness that thereby allows triggers (e.g. exercise) that would not narrow the airways to do so. But inflammation may also directly lead to an increase in asthma symptoms, such as cough and chest tightness, by activation of airway sensory nerve endings (**Figure 2**).

Although most attention has been focused on the acute inflammatory changes seen in asthmatic airways, it is apparent that asthma is a *chronic* inflammatory disease, with inflammation persisting over many years in most patients. Superimposed on this chronic inflammatory state are acute inflammatory episodes that correspond to exacerbation of asthma (**Figure 3**). It is clearly important to understand the mechanisms of acute and chronic inflammation in asthmatic airways and to investigate the effects of this chronic inflammation on airway function. It is

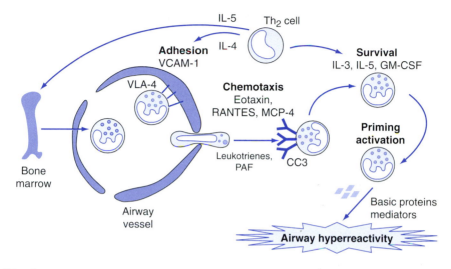

Figure 4
Eosinophilic inflammation in asthma. Eosinophils are derived in the bone marrow under the influence of IL-5, then adhere to the bronchial circulation, are recruited into the airway under the influence of chemotactic factors, survive in the airway and then are primed and activated to release mediators that contribute to airway hyperreactivity

also important to consider the effects of therapy on this inflammatory process.

Inflammatory cells

Many different inflammatory cells are involved in asthma and while no single inflammatory cell is able to account for the complex pathophysiology of asthma, some cells are predominant in asthmatic inflammation.

Mast cells: important in initiating the acute bronchoconstrictor response to allergen and probably to other indirect stimuli, such as exercise and hyperventilation (via osmolality of thermal changes) and fog.

Macrophages: may be activated by allergen via low affinity IgE receptors and may be important for initiating chronic inflammatory responses.

Dendritic cells: are the antigen-presenting cells of the airways and after ingesting allergen, migrate from the epithelium to regional lymph nodes where they programme the proliferation of T-lymphocytes.

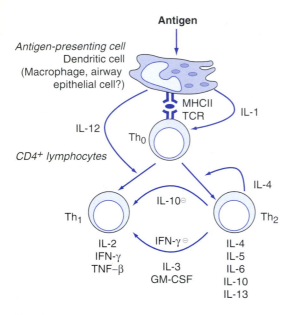

Antigen

Antigen-presenting cell
Dendritic cell
(Macrophage, airway
epithelial cell?)

MHCII
TCR

IL-1

IL-12

Th₀

CD4⁺ lymphocytes

IL-4

Th₁

IL-10⊖

Th₂

IL-2
IFN-γ
TNF–β

IFN-γ⊖

IL-3
GM-CSF

IL-4
IL-5
IL-6
IL-10
IL-13

Figure 5
Asthma is characterized by a preponderance of Th₂-helper T-cells over Th₁ cells

Eosinophils: are key inflammatory cells in asthma (*'chronic eosinophilic bronchitis'*) and are associated with AHR. They are recruited from the circulation via expression of adhesion molecules in the bronchial circulation and chemotactic factors in the airway (**Figure 4**). They are activated in the airways and release leukotrienes, oxygen-derived free radicals and basic proteins that may shed epithelial cells.

Lymphocytes: B-lymphocytes are involved in the synthesis of IgE, whereas T-lymphocytes orchestrate the eosinophilic inflammation. Dendritic cells programme the production of a T-helper (CD4⁺), cells (Th₂ cells) that secrete certain cytokines (IL-4 and IL-5) involved in eosinophil recruitment (**Figure 5**). There appears to be an imbalance of Th cells in allergy with the balance tipped in favour of Th₂ cells (**Figure 6**).

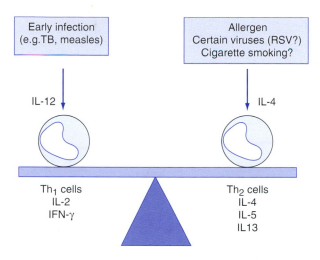

Figure 6
In allergic diseases there appears to be an imbalance between Th₁ and Th₂ cells, with the balance tipped in favour of Th₂ cells. Environmental factors, especially those operating in early life, may determine this imbalance

Neutrophils: do not appear to play a role in chronic asthma, but may be involved in acute exacerbations.

Structural cells: an important new concept in asthma is that structural cells within the airway wall are a source of inflammatory mediators and may orchestrate the inflammatory response. Airway epithelial cells may be an important source of inflammatory mediators and cytokines in asthma (**Figure 7**). Recent evidence suggests that proliferating airway smooth muscle may also release inflammatory mediators.

Inflammatory mediators

Many inflammatory mediators have been implicated in asthma and they may have a variety of effects on the airways that account for the pathological features of asthma. Mediators such as histamine, prostaglandins and leukotrienes contract airway smooth muscle, increase microvascular leakage, increase airway mucus secretion and

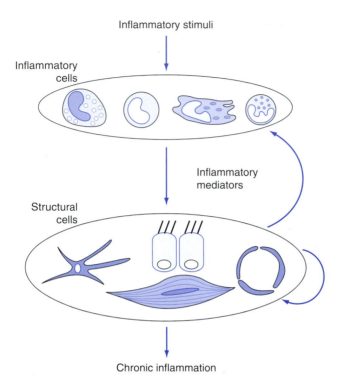

Inflammatory stimuli

Inflammatory
cells

Inflammatory
mediators

Structural
cells

Chronic inflammation

Figure 7
Structural cells in the airways (epithelial cells, airway smooth muscle cells, fibroblasts and endothelial cells) may be activated by inflammatory cells and mediators to themselves produce mediators that become an important mechanism for driving the chronic inflammatory process

attract other inflammatory cells (**Figure 8**). Because each mediator has many effects, the role of individual mediators in the pathophysiology of asthma is not yet clear. Indeed the multiplicity of mediators makes it unlikely that antago-nizing a single mediator will have a major impact on clinical asthma.

The cysteinyl-leukotrienes LTC_4, LTD_4 and LTE_4 are potent constrictors of human airways and both LTD_4 and LTE_4

Mediators and asthma

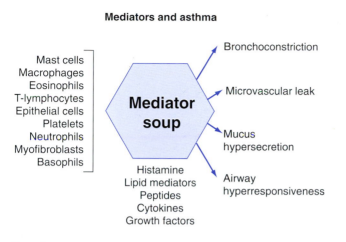

Mast cells
Macrophages
Eosinophils
T-lymphocytes
Epithelial cells
Platelets
Neutrophils
Myofibroblasts
Basophils

Mediator soup

Histamine
Lipid mediators
Peptides
Cytokines
Growth factors

Bronchoconstriction

Microvascular leak

Mucus hypersecretion

Airway hyperresponsiveness

Figure 8
There are multiple mediators involved in asthma and almost every cell in the airway may contribute to the complex mediator 'soup'. This mixture of mediators then produces the pathophysiology of asthma

increase airway hyperresponsiveness and may play an important role in asthma. The development of potent specific leukotriene antagonists and synthesis inhibitors have recently made it possible to evaluate the role of these mediators in asthma (see below). Anti-leukotrienes block allergen- and exercise-induced bronchoconstriction by approximately 50% and aspirin-induced bronchoconstriction in aspirin-sensitive asthmatic subjects by 100%. As discussed later, these drugs also have useful clinical effects in chronic asthma.

Platelet-activating factor (PAF) mimics many of the features of asthma, including airway hyperresponsiveness. However, potent PAF antagonists have proved to be disappointing in clinical trials of patients with chronic asthma.

Other mediators implicated in asthma include histamine, bradykinin, adenosine, reactive oxygen species, nitric oxide (NO) and endothelins. Inhibitors to all these mediators have now been developed, making it possible to evaluate their role in the pathophysiology of asthma.

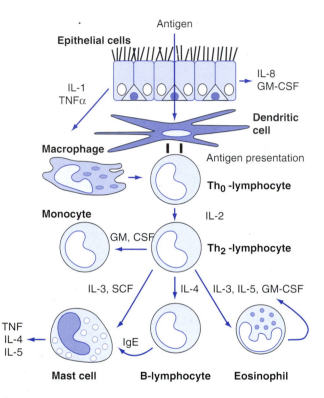

Figure 9
The cytokine network in asthma. Many inflammatory cytokines are released from inflammatory and structural cells in the airway and orchestrate and perpetuate the inflammatory response

Cytokines

Cytokines are increasingly recognized to be important in chronic inflammation and play a critical role in orchestrating the type of inflammatory response. Many inflammatory cells (macrophages, mast cells, eosinophils, lymphocytes) are capable of synthesizing and releasing these peptides, and structural cells (epithelial cells, airway smooth muscle cells, mast cells) may also release a variety of cytokines and may participate in the chronic inflammatory response (**Figure** 9). While inflammatory mediators like histamine and leukotrienes may be important in the acute and subacute inflammatory responses and in exacerbations of asthma, it is likely that cytokines play a dominant role in chronic inflammation. Every cell is capable of producing cytokines under certain conditions. Research in this area is hampered by a lack of specific antagonists although important observations have been made using specific neutralizing antibodies. The cytokines that appear to be of particular importance in asthma include the lymphokines secreted by T-lymphocytes: IL-3, which is important for the survival of mast cells in tissues; IL-4, which is critical in switching B-lymphocytes to produce IgE and for expression of VCAM-1 on endothelial cells; and IL-5, which is of critical importance in the differentiation, survival and priming of eosinophils. There is increased expression of IL-5 in lymphocytes in bronchial biopsies of patients with symptomatic asthma. Other cytokines, such as IL-1β, IL-6, IL-11, tumour necrosis factor-α (TNF-α) and GM-CSF are released from a variety of cells, including macrophages and epithelial cells, and may be important in amplifying the inflammatory response in asthma.

Chemokines are cytokines that have a chemotactic function. Two major classes of chemokine are recognized. CXC chemokines include IL-8 and predominantly attract neutrophils, whereas C-C chemokines attract lymphocytes, monocytes and eosinophils. Chemokines that are selective for eosinophil recruitment include RANTES, MCP-3, MCP-4 and eotaxin.

Some cytokines have *anti-inflammatory* effects and may modulate the inflammatory response in asthma. Interferon-γ (IFN-γ) and IL-12 inhibit Th$_2$ cells, whereas IL-10 inhibits the expression of multiple inflammatory cytokines and chemokines.

It is clear that no single mediator can be responsible for all the features of asthma, and it is likely that multiple mediators constitute an 'inflammatory soup' that may vary from patient to patient, depending on the relative state of activation of the different inflammatory cells. There may be important interactions between the different mediators and the concept of 'priming' may be very important because a combination of mediators may have a much greater effect than each mediator alone. This may be particularly important in the actions of cytokines, which

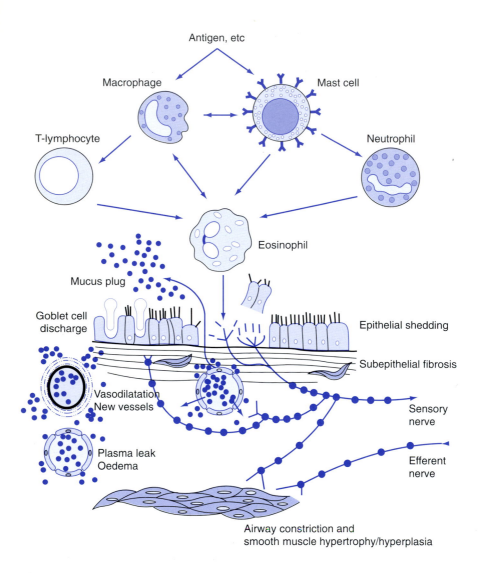

Figure 10
The pathophysiology of asthma is complex with participation of several interacting inflammatory cells, that result in acute and chronic inflammatory effects on the airway

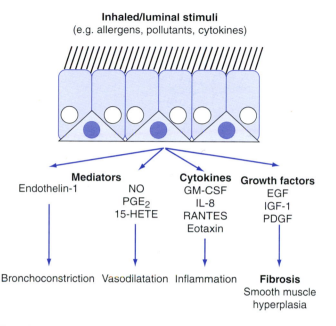

Inhaled/luminal stimuli
(e.g. allergens, pollutants, cytokines)

Mediators		**Cytokines**	**Growth factors**
Endothelin-1	NO	GM-CSF	EGF
	PGE_2	IL-8	IGF-1
	15-HETE	RANTES	PDGF
		Eotaxin	

Bronchoconstriction   Vasodilatation   Inflammation   **Fibrosis**
Smooth muscle
hyperplasia

Figure 11
Airway epithelial cells may play an active role in asthmatic inflammation through the release of many inflammatory mediators and cytokines

may have no effect in isolation, but may have a very pronounced effect after a cell has been exposed to another cytokine.

Inflammatory responses

The inflammatory response has several effects on the target cells of the airways, resulting in the characteristic pathophysiological changes associated with asthma (**Figure 10**).

Airway epithelium

Airway epithelium may be fragile in asthma as a result of the inflammatory process and this makes it prone to be shed. Epithelial cells are commonly found in clumps in the broncho-alveolar lavage (BAL) fluid or sputum (Creola bodies) of asthmatics, suggesting that there has been a loss of attachment to the basal layer or basement membrane. Epithelial cells themselves also produce inflammatory mediators (**Figure 11**), including multiple chemokines, cytokines, endothelin and growth factors.

Fibrosis

Electron microscopy of bronchial biopsies in asthmatic patients demonstrates that this thickening is due to subepithelial fibrosis due to the deposition of collagen fibres by myofibroblasts in the submucosal region. The subepithelial fibrosis may be one of the factors that contributes to the irreversible airway obstruction and the persisting airway hyperresponsiveness after corticosteroid treatment. This latter feature may be present even in mild asthmatics however.

Airway smooth muscle

There is still debate about the role of abnormalities in airway smooth muscle in asthmatic airways. In vitro airway smooth muscle from asthmatic patients usually shows no increased responsiveness to spasmogens, although exceptions are reported of increased maximal contractile effects or increased sensitivity to certain spasmogens. Reduced responsiveness to β-agonists has also been reported in post mortem or surgically removed bronchi from asthmatics, although the number of β-receptors is not reduced, suggesting that β-receptors have been uncoupled. These abnormalities of airway smooth muscle may be a reflection of the chronic inflammatory process. In asthmatic airways there is also a characteristic *hypertrophy* and *hyperplasia* of airway smooth muscle, which is presumably the result of stimulation of airway smooth muscle cells by various growth factors released from inflammatory cells.

Vascular responses

Vasodilatation occurs in inflammation, yet little is known about the role of the airway circulation in asthma, partly because of the difficulties involved in measuring airway blood flow. The bronchial circulation may play an important role in regulating airway calibre, since an increase in the vascular volume may contribute to airway narrowing. Passive venous congestion from left ventricular failure, results in increased airway reactivity to methacholine challenge.

Microvascular leakage is an essential component of the inflammatory response and many of the inflammatory mediators implicated in asthma produce this leakage. There is good evidence for microvascular leakage and plasma exudation in asthma and it may have several consequences on airway function, including increased airway secretions, impaired mucociliary clearance, formation of new mediators from plasma precursors (such as kinins) and mucosal oedema, all of which may contribute to airway narrowing and increased hyperresponsiveness.

Mucus secretion

Increased mucus secretion contributes to the viscid mucus plugs that occlude asthmatic airways, particularly in fatal asthma. There is evidence for hyperplasia of submucosal glands that are confined to large airways and of increased numbers of epithelial goblet cells. This increased secretory response may be due to inflammatory mediators acting on submucosal glands and due to stimulation of nerves. Little is understood about the control of goblet cells, which are the main source of mucus in peripheral airways, although recent studies investigating the control of goblet cells in guinea pig airways

suggest that cholinergic, adrenergic and sensory neuropeptides are important in stimulating secretion.

Nerves

Autonomic nervous control of the airways is complex, for, in addition to classical cholinergic and adrenergic mechanisms, non-adrenergic non-cholinergic (NANC) nerves and several neuropeptides have been identified in the respiratory tract. Many studies have investigated the possibility that defects in autonomic control may contribute to airway hyperresponsiveness and asthma, and abnormalities of autonomic function, such as enhanced cholinergic and α-adrenergic responses or reduced β-adrenergic responses, have been proposed. Current thinking suggests that these abnormalities are likely to be *secondary* to the disease, rather than primary defects. It is possible that airway inflammation may interact with autonomic control by several mechanisms.

Inflammatory mediators may act on various receptors on airway nerves to modulate the release of neurotransmitters. Thus, thromboxane enhances the release of acetylcholine from cholinergic nerves and thus exaggerates cholin-

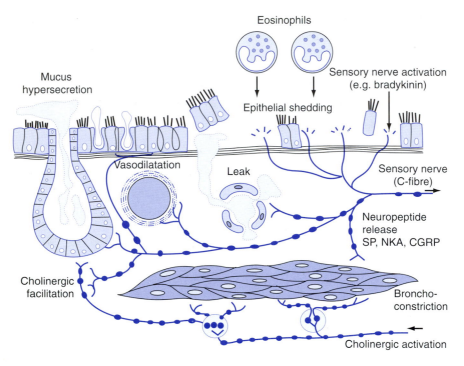

Figure 12
Neurogenic inflammation (axon reflex) in asthma may amplify inflammation through the release of neuropeptides such as substance P (SP), neurokinin A (NKA) and calcitonin gene-related peptide (CGRP) from airway sensory nerves

ergic bronchoconstriction. Inflammatory mediators may also activate sensory nerves, resulting in reflex cholinergic bronchoconstriction or release of inflammatory neuropeptides. Inflammatory products may also sensitize sensory nerve endings in the airway epithelium, so that the nerves become hyperalgesic. Hyperalgesia and pain (*dolor*) are cardinal signs of inflammation, and in the asthmatic airway may mediate cough and dyspnoea, which are such characteristic symptoms of asthma. The precise mechanisms of hyperalgesia are not yet certain, but mediators such as prostaglandins, bradykinin and certain cytokines may be important.

Bronchodilator nerves that are non-adrenergic are prominent in human airways, and it has been suggested that these nerves may be defective in asthma. In animal airways vasoactive intestinal peptide (VIP) has been shown to be a neurotransmitter of these nerves and a striking absence of VIP-immunoreactive nerves has been reported in the lungs from patients with severe fatal asthma. However, it is likely that this loss of VIP immunoreactivity is due to degradation by tryptase released from degranulating mast cells in the airways of asthmatics. In human airways the bronchodilator neurotransmitter appears to be nitric oxide.

Airway nerves may also release neurotransmitters that have inflammatory effects. Thus neuropeptides such as substance P (SP), neurokinin A and calcitonin-gene-related peptide may be released from sensitized inflammatory nerves in the airways that increase and extend the ongoing inflammatory response (neurogenic inflammation) (**Figure 12**). Although neurogenic inflammation is prominent in rodent models of asthma, there is, so far, little evidence that it is important in asthma.

Irreversible airway narrowing

Chronic inflammation in asthma may result in irreversible changes in airway structure that may result in irreversible airway obstruction. These changes include increased thickness of airway smooth muscle, fibrosis (which is predominantly subepithelial), increased numbers of mucus secreting cells and increased numbers of blood vessels (angiogenesis). These changes may not be reversible with therapy and may account for the accelerated annual decline in lung function. This may occur in some patients to a greater extent than others and may be increased by other factors such as concomitant cigarette smoking.

Transcription factors

Asthma is characterized by the expression of multiple inflammatory proteins (enzymes, cytokines, adhesion molecules, receptors) that are the result of increased gene expression. The induction of inflammatory genes is under the control of transcription factors, such as *activator protein-1* (AP-1) and *nuclear factor-κB* (NF-κB). NF-κB is of particular interest as it regulates the expression of many genes that are induced in asthma and may

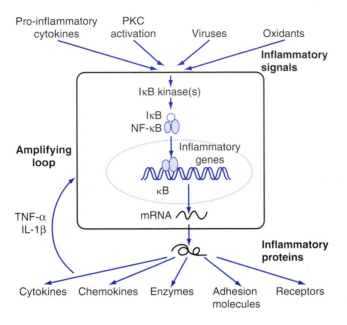

Figure 13
The transcription factor NF-κB may play a critical role in co-ordinating the expression of multiple inflammatory genes in asthmatic airway cells. Many inflammatory stimuli may be activated by NF-κB and this transcription factor is inhibited by corticosteroids

play a pivotal role in the amplification of the inflammatory process in asthma. NF-κB and AP-1 may also be targets for inhibition by glucocorticoids and may be important new therapeutic targets for the development of novel anti-inflammatory drugs (**Figure 13**). Many cytokines that are involved in asthma signal via the JAK-STAT transduction system (Janus kinase-signal transduc-tion-activated transcription factor), and STAT proteins may also be the target for the development of new drugs. Thus IL-4 and IL-13 signal through the unique STAT-6 transcription factor.

Genetics of asthma

There has been considerable interest in the genetics of asthma, particularly

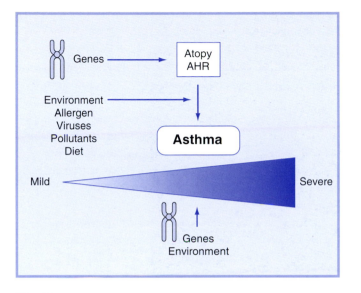

Figure 14
There is an interaction between genetic and environmental factors in asthma

from the point of view of understanding the causes of the disease and in identifying important therapeutic targets. There is clearly a familial tendency in asthma, with a concordance of approximately 30% in identical twins. Atopy is an inherited trait and several genes have been associated with the atopic status. These include the high affinity IgE β-receptor chain on chromosome 11q, the IL-4, IL-5, GM-CSF, IL-9 cluster of genes on 5q and the IL-4 receptor (α-chain). While the genetics of atopy are being elucidated, it is much less certain whether genetic factors are important in converting an atopic individual into an asthmatic patient. It is more likely that environmental factors, such as early allergen exposure and virus infections may be important in this respect. However, genetic factors are likely to be important in determining the severity of asthma and its response to different treatments (**Figure 14**). Thus two major polymorphisms of the β_2-adrenoceptor gene have been identified that result in variants of the β_2-receptor. An arginine→glycine substitution at codon 16 is associated with an increased tendency for downregulation of the receptor and an increased frequency for nocturnal asthma, whereas a glutamine→glutamic acid change at codon 27 is associated with reduced downregulation and a lesser degree of airway hyperresponsiveness. It is likely that many other polymorphisms affecting different genes involved in the inflammatory process will be identified in the future and associated with different phenotypic variants of asthma.

Monitoring inflammation in asthma

Since inflammation of the airways underlies the clinical features of asthma and an important goal of therapy is to suppress or prevent this inflammatory response. There have been considerable efforts to measure inflammation, preferably by non-invasive measurements that can be repeated and are relevant in the clinic. In research, bronchial biopsy and BAL by fibreoptic bronchoscopy has been extensively used to characterize the inflammatory process in asthma, but such techniques are invasive and obviously unsuited to routine clinical practice. Several approaches have been made:

Induced sputum: this is a research tool that is less invasive than bronchoscopy, but is time consuming and probably not suited to clinical practice. The advantage of the technique is that it is reasonably well tolerated by patients, and gives information about inflammatory cells and mediators in the airways.

Eosinophil cationic protein (ECP): this eosinophil granule protein can be measured in the blood, but does not correlate closely with asthma control. Sputum ECP may be more accurate.

Urinary LTE$_4$: measures the production of leukotrienes, but requires a complex assay.

Exhaled mediators: NO is formed in inflamed airways and can be detected in exhaled air by a chemiluminescence analyser. The levels are increased in patients with untreated asthma but are reduced by inhaled corticosteroid treatment (**Figure 15**). Exhaled carbon monoxide, another product of the inflammatory response, is also increased in patients with asthma (but may also be affected by cigarette smoking).

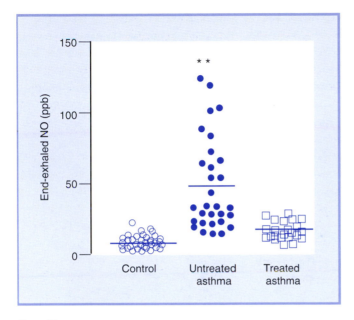

Figure 15
Exhaled nitric oxide (NO) is increased in untreated asthmatic patients compared with normal control subjects, but is reduced when asthma is treated with inhaled corticosteroids. Exhaled NO may be measured by a completely non-invasive method using a specially designed analyser

Rationale for therapy

The recognition that asthma is due to a special type of inflammation in the airways has led to the earlier and more widespread use of anti-inflammatory treatments, rather than an emphasis on bronchodilators to relieve symptoms. Indeed treatment with β_2-agonists, which controls asthma symptoms without suppressing inflammation, is potentially hazardous. Inhaled corticosteroids are the most effective anti-inflammatory drugs available and suppress most aspects of the inflammatory process, with effects on eosinophils, macrophages, T-lymphocytes, dendritic cells, mast cells and structural cells such as epithelial cells, which are a major source of inflammatory mediators in asthma. Since many mediators are involved in asthmatic inflammation it would seem unlikely that blocking a single mediator, such as histamine would be very useful in therapy. However, anti-leukotrienes do appear to have a useful clinical effect in many patients, indicating that cysteinyl-leukotrienes are predominant mediators and may have a useful place in therapy, particularly since cortico-steroids are not effective in blocking the synthesis of leukotrienes in asthma.

Asthma is an inflammatory disease that is localized to the airways and this provides an important rationale for therapy with inhaled drugs. Inhaled β_2-agonists are by far the most effective bronchodilators available, whereas inhaled corticosteroids are the most effective anti-inflammatory drugs. Furthermore, the inhaled route prevents or reduces the systemic side-effects of these drugs.

Better understanding of the mechanisms of asthma has allowed us to understand how currently used drugs work at a cellular and molecular level and this has led to more rationale use of these drugs. Research has also identified new targets for drug therapy and several new classes of drug for asthma are now in clinical development.

Further reading

Barnes PJ (1996) Pathophysiology of asthma. *Br J Clin Pharmacol* **42:** 3–10.

Barnes PJ, Grunstein MM, Leff AR and Woolcock AJ (1997) *Asthma.* Philadelphia: Lippincott–Raven, pp. 1–2183.

Barnes PJ, Chung KF and Page CP (1998) Inflammatory mediators of asthma: an update. *Pharmacol Rev* (in press).

Holgate ST (1997) Cellular and mediator basis of asthma in relationship to natural history. *Lancet* **350**(Suppl 2): S115–19.

Sandford A, Weir T and Pare P (1996) The genetics of asthma. *Am J Respir Crit Care Med* **153:** 1749–65.

Bronchodilators

2

Bronchodilator drugs have an 'anti-bronchoconstrictor' effect, which may be demonstrated directly in vitro by a relaxant effect on precontracted airways. Bronchodilators cause immediate reversal of airway obstruction in asthma in vivo, and this is believed to be due to an effect on airway smooth muscle, although additional pharmacological effects on other airway cells (such as reduced microvascular leakage and reduced release of bronchoconstrictor mediators from inflammatory cells) may contribute to the reduction in airway narrowing.

Three types of bronchodilator are in current clinical use:

- β-Adrenergic agonists (sympathomimetics)
- Methylxanthines (theophylline)
- Anticholinergics

Drugs such as cromoglycate, which prevent bronchoconstriction, have no direct bronchodilator action and are ineffective once bronchoconstriction

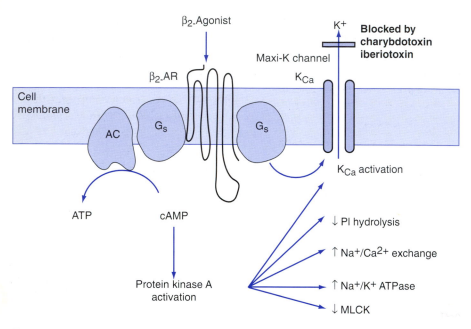

Figure 16
Molecular mechanisms involved in bronchodilator response to β_2-agonists. Activation of β_2-adrenoceptors (β_2AR) on airway smooth muscle cells is coupled via a G-protein (G_s) to adenyl cyclase (AC), resulting in increased intracellular cAMP formation. This activates protein kinase A which phosphorylates a number of substrates, including large conductance calcium-activated potassium channels (K_{Ca}), which can also be directly coupled to β_2-receptors

has occurred. Corticosteroids, while gradually improving airway obstruction, have no direct effect on contraction of airway smooth muscle and are not therefore considered to be bronchodilators.

β_2-Agonists

Inhaled β_2-agonists are the bronchodilator treatment of choice as they are the most effective bronchodilators and have minimal side-effects when used correctly. There is no place for short-acting and non-selective β_2-agonists such as isoprenaline and orciprenaline.

Mode of action

β_2-Agonists produce bronchodilatation by directly stimulating β_2-receptors in airway smooth muscle, which leads to relaxation. This can be demonstrated in vitro by the relaxant effect of isoprenaline on human bronchi and lung strips (indicating an effect of peripheral airways) and in vivo by a rapid decrease in airway resistance. β_2-Receptors have been demonstrated in airway smooth muscle by direct receptor-binding techniques and autoradiographic studies indicate that β_2-receptors are localized to smooth muscle of all airways from trachea to terminal bronchioles.

Activation of β_2-receptors results in activation of adenylyl cyclase and an increase in intracellular cAMP (**Figure 16**). This results in activation of a specific kinase (protein kinase A) that phosphorylates several target proteins within the cell, leading to relaxation. These processes include:

- Lowering of intracellular calcium ion (Ca^{2+}) concentration by active removal of Ca^{2+} from the cell and into intracellular stores
- An inhibitory effect on phosphoinositide hydrolysis
- Direct inhibition of myosin light chain kinase
- Opening of a large conductance calcium-activated potassium channel

(K^+) that repolarizes the smooth muscle cell and may stimulate the sequestration of Ca^{2+} into intracellular stores.

Recently, it has become apparent that β_2-agonists may be directly coupled to K^+ and that relaxation of airway smooth muscle may occur independently of an increase in cAMP. β_2-Agonists act as *functional antagonists* and reverse bronchoconstriction irrespective of the contractile agent. This is an important property, since many bronchoconstrictor mechanisms (inflammatory mediators and neurotransmitters) are likely to be contributory in asthma.

β_2-Agonists may have additional effects on airways, and β_2-receptors are localized to several different airway cells (**Table 1 and Figure 17**):

- Inhibition of *mediator release* from mast cells and other inflammatory cells
- Reduction and prevention of *microvascular leakage* and thus the development of bronchial mucosal oedema after exposure to mediators such as histamine and leukotrienes
- Increased *mucus secretion* from submucosal glands and ion trans-

Table 1
Localization and function of airway β_2-adrenoceptors.

Cell type	Subtype	Function
Smooth muscle	β_2	Relaxation (proximal distal)
		Inhibition of proliferation
Epithelium	β_2	Increased ion transport
		Secretion of inhibitory factor?
		Increased ciliary beating
		Increased mucociliary clearance
Submucosal glands	β_1/β_2	Increased secretion (mucus cells)
Clara cells	β_2	Increased secretion
Cholinergic nerves	β_2	Reduced acetylcholine release
Sensory nerves	β_2/β_3	Reduced neuropeptide release
		Reduced activation?
Bronchial vessels	β_2	Vasodilatation
		Reduced plasma extravasation
Inflammatory cells		
Mast cells	β_2	Reduced mediator release
Macrophages	β_2	No effect?
Eosinophils	β_2	Reduced mediator release
T-lymphocytes	β_2	Reduced cytokine release

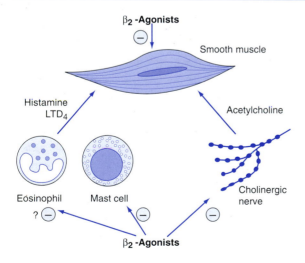

Figure 17
β_2-agonists may cause bronchodilatation directly via activation of β_2-receptors on airway smooth muscle, and also indirectly via inhibition of mediator release from inflammatory cells and neurotransmitter release from nerve endings

port across airway epithelium; these effects may enhance muco-ciliary clearance, and therefore reverse the defect in clearance found in asthma

- Reduction in *neurotransmission* in airway cholinergic nerves thus reducing cholinergic reflex bronchoconstriction
- Inhibition of the release of bronchoconstrictor and inflammatory peptides such as substance P from sensory nerves.

Although these additional effects of β_2-agonists may be relevant to the prophylactic use of these drugs against various challenges, their rapid bronchodilator action can probably be attributed to a direct effect on airway smooth muscle.

Anti-inflammatory effects?

Whether β_2-agonists have anti-inflammatory effects in asthma has become an important issue, particularly with their increasing use and the introduction of long-acting inhaled β_2-agonists. The inhibitory effects of β_2-agonists on mast-cell mediator release and microvascular leakage are clearly anti-inflammatory, suggesting that β_2-agonists may modify *acute* inflammation. However β_2-agonists do not appear to have a

significant inhibitory effect on the *chronic* inflammation of asthmatic airways that is controlled by corticosteroids. This has now been confirmed by biopsy studies in patients with asthma who are taking regular β_2-agonists that demonstrate no significant reduction in the number or activation in inflammatory cells in the airways, in contrast to the resolution of the inflammation that occurs with inhaled corticosteroids. This is likely to be related to the fact that β_2-agonists do not have an important inhibitory effect on macrophages, eosinophils or lymphocytes.

Current use

Short-acting inhaled β_2-agonists (such as salbutamol and terbutaline) are the most widely used and effective bronchodilators in the treatment of asthma. When inhaled from metered-dose aerosols they are convenient, easy to use, rapid in onset and without significant side-effects. In addition to an acute bronchodilator effect, they are effective in protecting against various challenges, such as exercise, cold air and allergen. They are the bronchodilators of choice in treating acute severe asthma, when the nebulized route of administration is as effective as intravenous use. The inhaled route of administration is preferable to the oral route because side-effects are fewer, and it may be more effective. Short-acting inhaled β_2-agonists should not be used on a regular basis in the treatment of mild asthma, but should be used as required by symptoms, since increased usage is then an indicator for the need for more anti-inflammatory therapy. Oral β_2-agonists are indicated as an additional bronchodilator. Slow-release preparations (such as slow-release salbutamol and bambuterol) may be indicated in nocturnal asthma, but are less useful than inhaled β_2-agonists because of an increased risk of side-effects. Long-acting inhaled β_2-agonists (salmeterol and formoterol) should be used as additional bronchodilators twice daily (see below).

Therapeutic choices

Several short-acting β_2-selective agonists are available (**Figure 18**). These drugs are as effective as non-selective agonists in their bronchodilator action, since airway effects are mediated only by β_2-receptors. However, they are less likely to produce cardiac stimulation than isoprenaline because β_1-receptors are stimulated relatively less. With the exception of rimiterol (which retains the catechol ring structure and is therefore susceptible to rapid metabolism), they have a longer duration of action because they are resistant to uptake and enzymatic degradation. There is little to choose between the various short-acting β-agonists currently available: all are usable by inhalation and orally, have a similar duration of action (usually 3–4 hours but less in severe asthma) and similar side-effects. Differences in β_2-selectivity have been claimed but are not clinically important. Drugs in clinical use include *salbutamol, terbutaline, fenoterol, tulobuterol, rimiterol* and *pirbuterol*. It has been claimed that fenoterol is less β_2-selective than salbutamol and terbutaline, resulting in increased cardiovascular side-effects, but this evidence is controversial, since all of these effects are mediated via β_2-receptors. The increased incidence of cardiovascular effects is more likely to be related to the greater effective dose of fenoterol and perhaps to more rapid absorption into the circulation.

Side-effects

Unwanted effects are dose related and are due to stimulation of extra-pulmonary β_2-receptors. Side-effects are not common with inhaled therapy, but

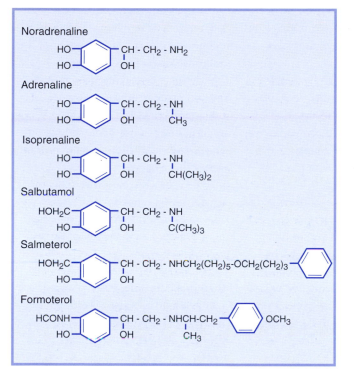

Figure 18
Structures of catecholamines showing the development of short- and long-acting selective β_2-agonists

more common with oral or intravenous administration.

- *Muscle tremor* due to stimulation of β_2-receptors in skeletal muscle is the commonest side-effect. It may be more troublesome with elderly patients

- *Tachycardia* and *palpitations* due to reflex cardiac stimulation secondary to peripheral vasodilatation, from direct stimulation of atrial β_2-receptors, and possibly also from stimulation of myocardial β_1-receptors as the doses of β_2-agonist are increased

- *Metabolic* effects (increase in free fatty acid, insulin, glucose, pyruvate and lactate) seen only after large systemic doses
- *Hypokalaemia* due to β_2-receptor stimulation of potassium entry into skeletal muscle. Hypokalaemia might be serious in the presence of hypoxia, as in acute asthma, when there may be a predisposition to cardiac dysrrhythmias
- Increased *ventilation-perfusion (V̇/Q̇) mismatching* by causing pulmonary vasodilatation in blood vessels previously constricted by hypoxia, resulting in the shunting of blood to poorly ventilated areas and a fall in arterial oxygen tension. Although in practice the effect of β-agonists on Pao_2 is usually very small (<5 mm Hg fall), occasionally in severe chronic airways obstruction it is large, although it may be prevented by giving additional inspired oxygen.

Tolerance

Continuous treatment with an agonist often leads to tolerance (subsensitivity, desensitization), which may be due to uncoupling and/or downregulation of the receptor. There have been many studies of bronchial β-receptor function after prolonged therapy with β-agonists. Tolerance of non-airway β-receptor responses, such as tremor and cardiovascular and metabolic responses, is readily induced in normal and asthmatic subjects. Tolerance of human airway smooth muscle to β-agonists in vitro has been demonstrated, although the concentration of agonist necessary is high and the degree of desensitization is variable. Animal studies suggest that airway smooth muscle β_2-receptors may be more resistant to desensitization than β_2-receptors elsewhere due to a high receptor reserve. In normal subjects bronchodilator tolerance has been demonstrated in some studies after high-dose inhaled salbutamol, but not in others. In asthmatic patients tolerance to the bronchodilator effects of β_2-agonists has not usually been found. However, tolerance develops to the bronchoprotective effects of β_2-agonists and this is more marked with indirect constrictors, such as adenosine, allergen and exercise, that activate mast cells than with direct constrictors such as histamine and methacholine (**Figure 19**). The high level of β_2-receptor gene expression in airway smooth muscle compared with peripheral lung may also contribute to the resistance to tolerance since there is likely to be a

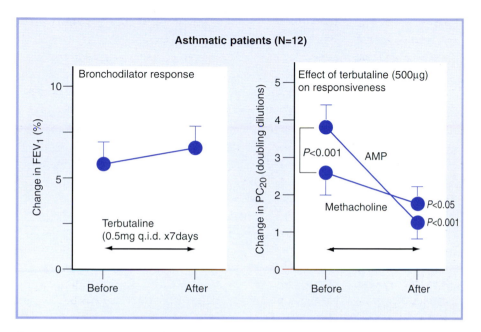

Figure 19

Development of tolerance to the protective effects of a short-acting inhaled β₂-agonist (terbutaline). After 1 week of regular treatment there is no loss of bronchodilator effect, but a significant loss of protection against bronchoconstriction induced by AMP and the cholinergic agonist and methacholine. The greater protective effect of AMP compared with methacholine represents a mast-cell inhibitory effect of the β₂-agonist and this study shows that the protective effect of AMP is lost to a greater extent than with methacholine challenge, indicating greater tolerance of β₂-agonists in mast cells than in airway smooth muscle cells. (Adapted from O'Connor et al (1992))

high rate of β-receptor synthesis. Tolerance to the bronchodilator effects of the long-acting β₂-agonist formoterol has been reported.

Experimental studies have shown that corticosteroids prevent the develop- ment of tolerance in airway smooth muscle, and prevent and reverse the fall in pulmonary β-receptor density. However, recent studies suggest that inhaled corticosteroids do not prevent tolerance to the bronchoprotective effect of inhaled β₂-agonists.

Safety

Because of a possible relationship between adrenergic drug therapy and the rise in asthma deaths in several countries during the early 1960s, doubts have been cast on the safety of β-agonists. A causal relationship between β-agonist use and mortality has never been established, although in retrospective studies this would not be possible. A particular $β_2$-agonist, fenoterol, has been linked to the rise in asthma deaths in New Zealand during the 1980s since significantly more of the fatal cases were prescribed fenoterol than the case-matched control patients. This association was strengthened by subsequent studies and by a fall in asthma mortality when fenoterol was withdrawn. An epidemiological study based in Saskatchewan, Canada, examined the links between drugs prescribed for asthma and death or near death from asthma attacks, based on computerized records of prescriptions. There was a marked increase in the risk of death with high doses of all inhaled β-agonists. The risk was greater with fenoterol, but when the dose was adjusted to the equivalent dose for salbutamol there was no significant difference in the risk of these two drugs. The link between high-dose β-agonist usage and increased asthma mortality does not prove a causal association, since patients with more severe and poorly controlled asthma, and who are therefore more likely to have an increased risk of fatal attacks, are more likely to be using higher doses of β-agonist inhalers and less likely to be using effective anti-inflammatory treatment. Indeed in the patients who used regular inhaled corticosteroids there was a significant reduction in risk of death.

Regular use of inhaled β-agonists may increase asthma *morbidity*. In a study carried out in New Zealand the regular use of fenoterol was associated with poorer control and a small increase in airway hyperresponsiveness compared with patients using fenoterol 'on demand' for symptom control over a 6-month period. However this was not found in studies with salbutamol, although a small increase in airway hyperresponsiveness has been found. There is some evidence that regular inhaled salbutamol may increase exercise-induced asthma and increase inflammation in asthmatic airways. One possible mechanism is that β-agonists may inhibit the anti-inflammatory action of glucocorticoids.

While it is unlikely that normally recommended doses of β_2-agonists worsen asthma, it is possible that this could occur with larger doses. Furthermore, some patients may be particularly susceptible if they have polymorphisms of the β_2-receptor that more rapidly downregulate. Short-acting inhaled β_2-agonists should only be used 'on demand' for symptom control and if they are required frequently (more than three times weekly) then an inhaled anti-inflammatory drug is indicated. There is an association between increased risk of death from asthma and the use of high doses of inhaled β_2-agonists; while this may reflect severity, it is also possible that high-dose β_2-agonists may have a deleterious effect on asthma. High concentrations of β_2-agonists interfere with the anti-inflammatory action of corticosteroids. Patients on high doses of β_2-agonists (> 1 canister per month) should be treated with effective anti-inflammatory treatments and attempts should be made to reduce the daily dose of inhaled β_2-agonist.

Long-acting inhaled β_2-agonists

The long-acting inhaled β_2-agonists salmeterol and formoterol have been a major advance in asthma therapy. Both drugs have a bronchodilator action of more than 12 hours and also protect against bronchoconstriction for a similar period. They are particularly useful in treating nocturnal asthma. Both improve asthma control (when given twice daily) compared with regular treatment with short-acting β_2-agonists four times daily (**Figure 20**). Both drugs are well tolerated. Tolerance to the bronchodilator effect of formoterol and the bronchoprotective effects of formoterol and salmeterol have been demonstrated, but this is not a loss of protection, does not appear to be progressive and is of doubtful clinical significance. While both drugs have a similar duration of effect in clinical studies there are some differences. Formoterol has a more rapid onset of action and is a fuller agonist than salmeterol. This might confer a theoretical advantage in more severe asthma, whereas it may also make it more likely to induce tolerance. Studies comparing the clinical efficacy of both drugs in mild and severe asthmatic patients are now needed.

Recent studies have suggested that inhaled long-acting β_2-agonists might be introduced earlier in therapy. In

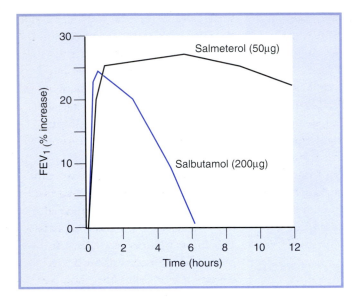

Figure 20
The inhaled long-acting β_2-agonist salmeterol, has a much longer duration of bronchodilator action than salbutamol

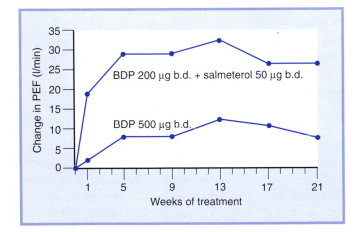

Figure 21
In patients not controlled on beclomethasone dipropionate (BDP) 400 µg daily, addition of the long-acting inhaled β_2-agonist salmeterol has a better effect than increasing the dose of inhaled corticosteroid. (Adapted from Greening et al (1994))

asthmatic patients not controlled on either 400 or 800 µg inhaled cortico-steroids, addition of salmeterol gives better control of asthma than increasing the dose of inhaled corticosteroid (**Figure 21**). This has also been found with formoterol, which has in addition been shown to reduce the frequency of asthma exacerbations. This suggests that long-acting inhaled β_2-agonists may be added to low-dose inhaled cortico-steroids if asthma is not controlled, as an alternative (and perhaps in preference) to increasing the dose of inhaled corticosteroids.

At present it is recommended that long-acting inhaled β_2-agonists should only be used in patients who are also prescribed inhaled corticosteroids. In the future, long-acting inhaled β_2-agonists may be used with cortico-steroids in fixed combination inhalers (formoterol + budesonide, salmeterol + fluticasone) in order to improve compliance and reduce the risk of patients using these drugs as sole long-term treatment.

Theophylline

Methylxanthines such as theophylline, which are related to caffeine, have been used in the treatment of asthma since 1930. Indeed, theophylline is still the most widely used anti-asthma therapy world-wide because it is inexpensive. Theophylline became more useful with the availability of rapid plasma assays and the introduction of reliable slow-release preparations. However, the frequency of side-effects and the relative low efficacy of theophylline have recently led to reduced usage since β_2-agonists are far more effective as bronchodilators and inhaled corticosteroids have a greater anti-inflammatory effect. In patients with severe asthma it still remains a very useful drug, however. There is increasing evidence that theophylline has an anti-inflammatory or immunomodulatory effect and may be effective in combination with inhaled corticosteroids.

Mode of action

Although theophylline has been in clinical use for more than 50 years its mechanism of action is still uncertain and several modes of action have been proposed (**Table 2**):

- *Inhibition of phosphodiesterases* (PDE), which break down cAMP in the cell, thereby leading to an increase in intracellular cAMP

Table 2
Mechanisms of action of theophylline.

- Phosphodiesterase inhibition
- Adenosine receptor antagonism
- Stimulation of catecholamine release
- Mediator inhibition
- Inhibition of intracellular calcium release

concentrations **(Figure 22)**. Theophylline is a non-selective PDE inhibitor, but the degree of

inhibition is minor at concentrations of theophylline that are within the 'therapeutic range'. This is likely to account for the bronchodilator action of theophylline

- *Adenosine receptor antagonism* since adenosine is a bronchoconstrictor in asthmatic patients through activation of mast cells. Enprofylline, which is more potent than theophylline as a bronchodilator, has no significant inhibitory effect on adenosine receptors at therapeutic concentrations, suggesting that

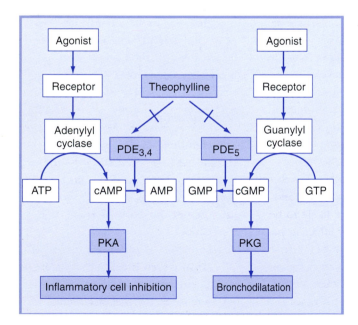

Figure 22
Theophylline is a weak phosphodiesterase (PDE) inhibitor, increasing the concentrations of cAMP and cGMP in airway cells, resulting in bronchodilatation and inhibition of inflammatory cells

adenosine antagonism is an unlikely explanation for the bronchodilator effect of theophylline. However, adenosine antagonism may account for some of the side-effects of theophylline, such as central nervous system stimulation, cardiac arrhythmias and diuresis

• Increased *secretion of adrenaline* from the adrenal medulla. However, the increase in plasma concentration is small and insufficient to account for any significant bronchodilator effect.

Despite extensive study, it has been difficult to elucidate the molecular mechanism for the bronchodilatation or other anti-asthma actions of theophylline. It is possible that any beneficial effect in asthma is related to its action on other cells (such as platelets, T-lymphocytes or macrophages) or on airway microvascular leak and oedema in addition to airway smooth muscle relaxation (**Figure 23**). Indeed theophylline is a rather ineffective bronchodilator and its anti-asthma effect is more likely to be explained by some other effect. It may be relevant that theophylline is ineffective when given by inhalation, but is effective when a critical plasma concentration is reached. This may

indicate that it is having important effects on cells other than those in the airway. It is possible that theophylline acts as an immunomodulator and has effects on T-lymphocyte function in vitro. A placebo-controlled theophylline withdrawal study indicates that theophylline appears to have an immunomodulatory effect and decreases the number of activated T-cells in the airways probably by blocking their trafficking from the circulation. Theophylline inhibits the late response to allergen challenge more effectively than the early response and inhibits the influx of eosinophils into the airways.

Clinical use

In patients with acute asthma intravenous aminophylline is less effective than nebulized β_2-agonists, and should therefore be reserved for those patients who fail to respond to β_2-agonists. Theophylline should not be added routinely to nebulized β_2-agonists since it does not increase the bronchodilator response and may only increase their side-effects.

Theophylline has little or no effect on bronchomotor tone in normal airways, but reverses bronchoconstriction in

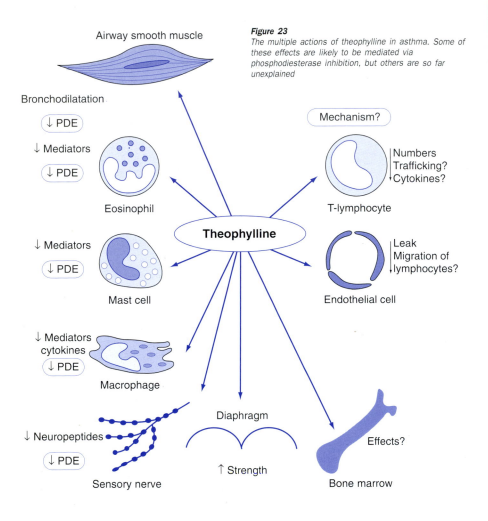

Figure 23
The multiple actions of theophylline in asthma. Some of these effects are likely to be mediated via phosphodiesterase inhibition, but others are so far unexplained

asthmatic patients, although it is less effective than inhaled β-agonists and is more likely to have unwanted effects. Theophylline and β-agonists have additive effects, even if true synergy is not seen, and there is evidence that theophylline may provide an additional bronchodilator effect even when maximally effective doses of β-agonist have been given. This means that, if

Table 3
Factors affecting clearance of theophylline.

Increased clearance
- Enzyme induction (rifampicin, phenobarbitone, ethanol)
- Smoking (tobacco, marijuana)
- High protein, low carbohydrate diet
- Barbecued meat
- Childhood

Decreased clearance
- Enzyme inhibition (crimetidine, erythromycin, ciprofloxacin, allopurinol, zileuton)
- Congestive heart failure
- Liver disease
- Pneumonia
- Viral infection and vaccination
- High carbohydrate diet
- Old age

adequate bronchodilatation is not achieved by a β-agonist alone, theophylline may be added to the maintenance therapy with benefit. Theophylline may be useful in some patients with nocturnal asthma, since slow-release preparations are able to provide therapeutic concentrations overnight and are more effective than slow-release β-agonists. Although theophylline is less effective than a β-agonist and corticosteroids there are some asthmatic patients who appear to derive unexpected benefit, and even patients on oral corticosteroids may show a deterioration in lung function when theophylline is withdrawn.

Recent studies suggest that addition of low-dose theophylline is as effective as doubling the dose of inhaled corticosteroids in patients not controlled on low doses of inhaled corticosteroids.

Theophylline is readily and reliably absorbed from the gastrointestinal tract, but there are many factors that effect plasma clearance, and therefore plasma concentration, which make the drug relatively difficult to use (**Table 3**).

There are many different formulations of slow-release theophylline or aminophylline available and these differ in their pharmacokinetic profile. Several preparations are available for twice daily administration and there are also once daily preparations. Twice daily administration may be preferable with a higher dose given at night to prevent nocturnal bronchoconstriction, whereas a lower dose is needed in the day as inhaled β-agonists may be used as additional bronchodilators. This may reduce the frequency of side-effects. Caution should be observed when switching from one slow release preparation to another.

Recent studies suggest that low-dose theophylline (giving plasma concentrations of 5–10 mg/l) is effective in controlling asthma. This dose is below the previously recommended doses for theophylline based on plasma concentrations needed for bronchodilatation (10–20 mg/l) (**Figure 24**).

Side-effects

Unwanted effects of theophylline are usually related to plasma concentration and tend to occur when plasma levels

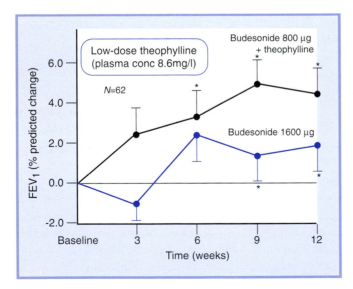

Figure 24
In patients not controlled on budesonide 400 µg daily, addition of low-dose theophylline has a better effect than doubling the dose of inhaled corticosteroid. (Adapted from Evans et al (1997))

Table 4
Side-effects of theophylline.

- Nausea and vomiting
- Headaches
- Gastric discomfort
- Diuresis
- Behavioural disturbance (?)
- Cardiac arrhythmias
- Epileptic seizures

exceed 20 mg/l. However, some patients develop side-effects even at low plasma concentrations. To some extent side-effects may be reduced by gradually increasing the dose until therapeutic concentrations are achieved.

The commonest side-effects are headache, nausea and vomiting, abdominal discomfort and restlessness (**Table** 4). There may also be increased acid secretion and diuresis. There was concern that theophylline, even at therapeutic concentrations, may lead to behavioural disturbance and learning difficulties in school children, but there is no convincing evidence for this.

At high concentrations convulsions and cardiac arrhythmias may occur. Some

of the side-effects (central stimulation, gastric secretion, diuresis and arrhythmias) may be due to adenosine receptor antagonism and may therefore be avoided by drugs such as enprofylline, which has no significant adenosine antagonism at bronchodilator doses.

Anticholinergics

Atropine, a naturally occurring compound, was also introduced for treating asthma but, because these compounds gave side-effects, particularly drying of secretions, less soluble quaternary compounds, such as atropine methylnitrate and ipratropium bromide, were introduced. These compounds are topically active and are not significantly absorbed from the respiratory tract or from the gastrointestinal tract.

Mode of action

Anticholinergics are specific antagonists of muscarinic receptors and inhibit cholinergic nerve-induced bronchoconstriction. There is a small degree of resting bronchomotor tone due to tonic cholinergic nerve impulses that release acetylcholine in the vicinity of airway smooth muscle and cholinergic reflex bronchoconstriction may be initiated by irritants, cold air and stress.

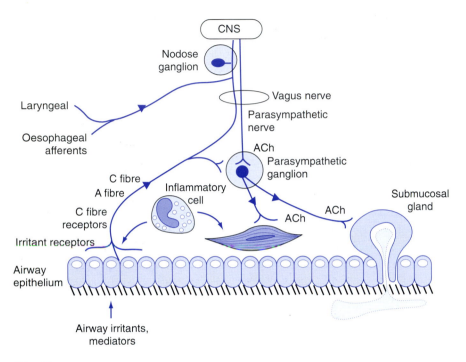

Figure 25
Cholinergic control of airway smooth muscle. Pre-ganglionic and post-ganglionic parasympathetic nerves release acetylcholine (ACh) and can be activated by airway and extrapulmonary afferent nerves. Note that mediators released from inflammatory cells directly activate airway smooth muscle cells, as well as activating a cholinergic reflex, so that anticholinergics are less effective than β_2-agonists as bronchodilators in asthma, since the latter counteract the effect of all bronchoconstrictors

While anticholinergics afford protection against acute challenge by sulphur dioxide, inert dusts, cold air and emotional factors, they are less effective against antigen challenge, exercise and fog. This is not surprising, as anticholinergic drugs will only inhibit reflex cholinergic bronchoconstriction and could have no significant blocking effect on the *direct* effects of inflammatory mediators such as histamine and leukotrienes on bronchial smooth muscle (**Figure 25**). Furthermore, cholinergic antagonists probably have little or no effect on mast cells, microvascular leak or the chronic inflammatory response. For these reasons anticholinergics are less effective as bronchodilators than β_2-agonists in patients with asthma.

Clinical use

In asthmatic subjects anticholinergic drugs are less effective as bronchodilators than β_2-agonists and offer less efficient protection against various bronchial challenges, although their duration of action is significantly longer. These drugs may be more effective in older patients with asthma in whom there is an element of fixed airway obstruction. Nebulized anticholinergic drugs are effective in acute severe asthma, although they are less effective than β_2-agonists in this situation. Nevertheless, in the acute and chronic treatment of asthma anticholinergic drugs may have an additive effect with β_2-agonists and should therefore be considered when control of asthma is not adequate with β_2-agonists, particularly if there are problems with theophylline, or inhaled β_2-agonists give troublesome tremor in elderly patients. The time course of bronchodilatation with anticholinergic drugs is slower than with β_2-agonists, reaching a peak only 1 h after inhalation, but persists for over 6 h.

In chronic obstructive pulmonary disease (COPD) anticholinergic drugs may be as effective as, or even superior to β_2-agonists. Their relatively greater effect in chronic obstructive airways disease than in asthma may be explained by an inhibitory effect on vagal tone which, while not necessarily being increased in COPD, may be the only reversible element of airway obstruction which is exaggerated by geometric factors in a narrowed airway (**Figure 26**).

Therapeutic choices

Ipratropium bromide is the most widely used anticholinergic inhaler and is available as a metered-dose inhaler (MDI) and a nebulized preparation. The onset of bronchodilatation is relatively slow and is usually maximal 30–60 min after inhalation, but may persist for up to 8 h. It is usually given by MDI three to four times daily on a regular basis, rather than intermittently for symptom relief, in view of its slow onset of action.

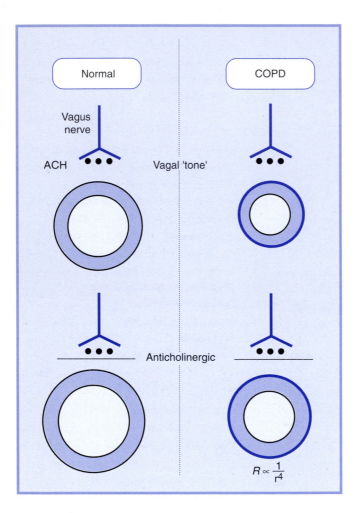

Normal

COPD

Vagus nerve

ACH

Vagal 'tone'

Anticholinergic

$$R \propto \frac{1}{r^4}$$

Figure 26
Cholinergic control of airways in patients with chronic obstructive pulmonary disease (COPD). Normal airways have a certain degree of vagal cholinergic tone due to tonic release of acetylcholine (ACh) that is blocked by muscarinic antagonists. This effect may be exaggerated in patients with COPD, because of fixed narrowing of the airways as a result of geometric factors. This predicts that anticholinergic drugs will have a greater bronchodilator effect in COPD than in normal airways

Oxitropium bromide is a quaternary anticholinergic bronchodilator that is similar to ipratropium bromide in terms of receptor blockade. It is available in higher doses by inhalation and may therefore have a more prolonged effect. Thus, it may be useful in some patients with nocturnal asthma.

Side-effects

Inhaled anticholinergic drugs are usually well tolerated and there is no evidence for any decline in responsiveness with continued use. On stopping inhaled anticholinergics a small rebound increase in responsiveness has been described, but the clinical relevance of this is uncertain. Atropine has side-effects that are dose related and are due to cholinergic antagonism in other systems and may lead to dryness of the mouth, blurred vision and urinary retention. Systemic side-effects after ipratropium bromide are very uncommon because there is virtually no systemic absorption. Because cholinergic agonists stimulate *mucus secretion* there have been several studies of mucus secretion with anticholinergic drugs as there has been concern that they may reduce secretion and lead to more viscous mucus. Atropine reduces mucociliary clearance in normal subjects and in patients with asthma and chronic bronchitis, but ipratropium bromide, even in high doses, has no detectable effect in either normal subjects or in patients with airway disease. A significant unwanted effect is the unpleasant *bitter* taste of inhaled ipratropium, which may contribute to poor compliance with this drug. Nebulized ipratropium bromide may precipitate *glaucoma* in elderly patients due to a direct effect of the nebulized drug on the eye. This may be prevented by nebulization with a mouth piece rather than a face mask.

Reports of *paradoxical bronchoconstriction* with ipratropium bromide, particularly when given by nebulizer, were largely explained by the hypotonicity of the nebulizer solution and by antibacterial additives, such as benzalkonium chloride and EDTA. Nebulizer solutions free of these problems are less likely to cause bronchoconstriction. Occasionally, bronchoconstriction may occur with ipratropium bromode given by MDI. It is possible that this is due to blockade of pre-junctional M_2-receptors on airway cholinergic nerves that normally inhibit acetylcholine release.

Further reading

Barnes PJ (1995) Beta-adrenergic receptors and their regulation. *Am J Respir Crit Care Med* **152:** 838–60.

Barnes PJ and Buist AS (1997) The role of anticholinergics in COPD and chronic asthma. London: Gardner Caldwell Publications, 1997; 1–172.

Barnes PJ and Pauwels RA (1994) Theophylline in asthma: time for reappraisal? *Eur Resp J* **7:** 579–91.

Boulet L (1994) Long versus short-acting β_2-agonists. *Drugs* **47:** 207–22.

Evans DJ, Taylor DA, Zetterstrom O et al (1997) A comparison of low-dose inhaled budesonide plus theophylline and high-dose inhaled budesonide for moderate asthma. *N Engl J Med* **337:** 1412–18.

Greening AP, Ind PW, Northfield M et al (1994) Added salmeterol versus higher-dose corticosteroid in asthma patients with symptoms on existing inhaled corticosteroid. *Lancet* **344:** 219–24.

Gross NJ (1992) Anticholinergic bronchodilators. In PJ Barnes, IW Rodger and NC Thomson, eds. *Asthma: Basic Mechanisms and Clinical Management,* 2nd edn. London: Academic Press, pp. 555–66.

Nelson HS (1995) Beta-adrenergic bronchodilators. *New Engl J Med* **333:** 499–506.

O'Connor BJ, Aikman SL and Barnes PJ (1992) Tolerance to the nonbronchodilator effects of inhaled β_2-agonists. *N Engl J Med* **327:** 1204–8.

Weinberger M and Hendeles L (1996) Theophylline in asthma. *New Engl J Med* **334:** 1380–8.

Corticosteroids

3

Corticosteroids were introduced for the treatment of asthma shortly after their discovery in the 1950s and remain the most effective therapy available for asthma. However, side-effects and fear of adverse effects have limited their use and there has therefore been considerable research into discovering new or related agents that retain the beneficial action on airways without unwanted effects. The introduction of inhaled corticosteroids has revolutionized the treatment of chronic asthma and now that asthma is viewed as a chronic inflammatory disease, inhaled corticosteroids may even be considered as first-line therapy in patients with chronic asthma.

Mode of action

Corticosteroids enter target cells and bind to cytosolic glucocorticoid receptors. There is only one type of glucocorticoid receptor and no evidence for different subtypes that might mediate different

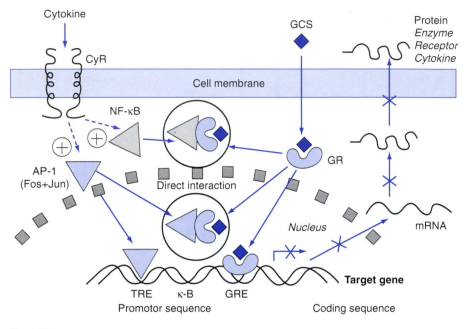

Figure 27
Direct interaction between the transcription factors activator protein-1 (AP-1) and nuclear factor-kappa B (NF-κB) and the glucocorticoid receptor (GR) may result in mutual repression. In this way steroids may counteract the chronic inflammatory effects of cytokines that activate these transcription factors

aspects of corticosteroid action. The steroid–receptor complex is transported to the nucleus where it binds to specific sequences on the upstream regulatory element of certain target genes, resulting in increased or decreased transcription of the gene that leads to increased or decreased protein synthesis. Glucocorticoid receptors may also interact *directly* with

protein transcription factors in the cytoplasm and thereby influence the synthesis of certain proteins independently of an interaction with DNA in the cell nucleus. The direct repression of transcription factors, such as AP-1 and NF-κB is likely to account for many of the anti-inflammatory effects of corticosteroids in asthma (**Figures 27 and 28**).

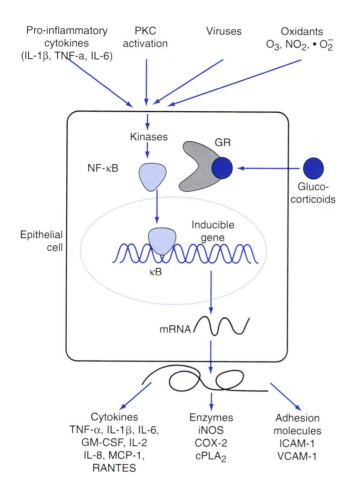

Figure 28
Inhibitory effect of corticosteroids on nuclear factor-κB (NF-κB), resulting in reduced expression of the multiple inflammatory genes that are switched on in asthma

The mechanism of action of corticosteroids in asthma is still poorly understood, but is most likely to be related to their anti-inflammatory properties. As discussed in Chapter 1, there is compelling evidence that asthma and airway hyerresponsiveness are due to an inflammatory process in the airways and there are several cells involved in this inflammatory response that might be inhibited by corticosteroids (**Figure 29**). Airway epithelial cells may be a particularly important target for inhaled corticosteroid action and suppression of mediator release from these surface cells may control inflammation within the airway wall (**Figure 30**). Several studies of bronchial biopsies in asthma

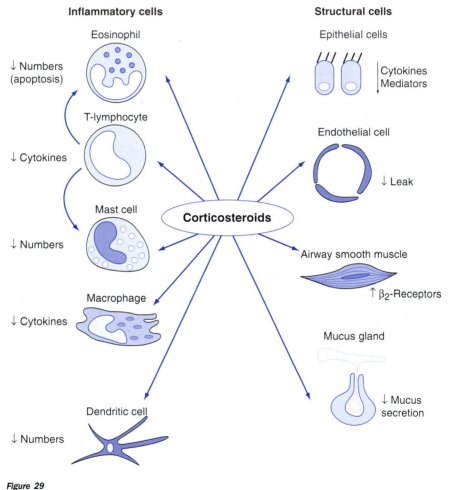

Figure 29
Cellular effect of corticosteroids

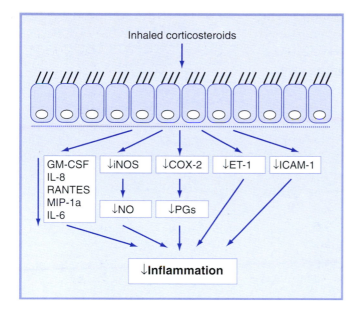

Figure 30
Inhaled corticosteroids may inhibit the transcription of several 'inflammatory' genes in airway epithelial cells and thus reduce inflammation in the airway wall

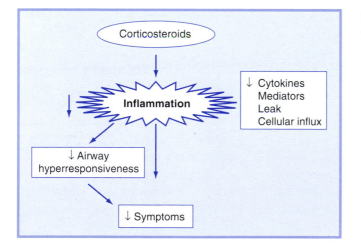

Figure 31
Corticosteroids suppress inflammation and therefore reduce airway hyperresponsiveness and symptoms

have demonstrated a reduction in the number and activation of inflammatory cells in the epithelium and submucosa after regular inhaled corticosteroids, together with a healing of the damaged epithelium. Indeed in mild asthmatics the inflammation may be completely resolved after inhaled corticosteroids. Suppression of inflammation then results in reduced airway hyper-responsiveness and symptoms (**Figure 31**).

Corticosteroids potently inhibit the formation of cytokines, such as IL-1, IL-2, IL-3, IL-4, IL-5, IL-13, GM-CSF by lymphocytes and macrophages (**Table 5**). Indeed this may be the most important action of corticosteroids in suppressing asthmatic inflammation, since cytokines may play a very critical role in the maintenance of the chronic eosinophilic inflammation.

Corticosteroids prevent and reverse the increase in vascular permeability due to inflammatory mediators in animal studies and may therefore lead to resolution of airway oedema. Corticosteroids also have a direct inhibitory effect on mucus glycoprotein secretion from airway submucosal glands, as well as indirect inhibitory effects by downregulation of inflammatory stimuli.

Table 5
Effect of corticosteroids on gene transcription.

Increased transcription
- Lipocortin-1
- 2-Adrenoceptor
- Secretory leukocyte inhibitory protein
- IκB-α (inhibitor of NF-κB)
- Anti-inflammatory cytokines
  IL-10, IL-12, IL-1 receptor antagonist

Decreased transcription
- Inflammatory cytokines
  IL-2, IL-3, IL-4, IL-5, IL-6, IL-8, IL-11, IL-13, TNF-α, GM-CSF, SCF
- Chemokines
  RANTES, MIP-1α, eotaxin

- Inducible nitric oxide synthase (iNOS)
- Inducible cyclo-oxygenase (COX-2)
- Inducible phospholipase A2 (cPLA2)
- Endothelin-1
- NK1-receptors
- Adhesion molecules (ICAM-1, VCAM-1)

Corticosteroids have no direct effect on contractile responses of airway smooth muscle and improvement in lung function is presumably due to an effect on the chronic airway inflammation and airway hyperresponsiveness. After a single dose, inhaled corticosteroids have no effect on the early response to allergen (reflecting their lack of effect on mast cell mediator release), but inhibit the late response (which may be due to an effect on macrophages and eosinophils) and also inhibit the increase in airway hyperresponsiveness. Inhaled corticosteroids also reduce airway hyperresponsiveness but this effect may take several weeks or months and presumably reflects the slow healing of the damaged inflamed airway.

It is important to recognize that corticosteroids *suppress* inflammation in the airways but do not cure the underlying disease. When corticosteroids are withdrawn there is a recurrence of the same degree of airway hyperresponsiveness, although in patients with mild asthma it may take several months to return.

·Corticosteroids increase β_2-adrenergic responsiveness, but whether this is relevant to their effect in asthma is uncertain. Corticosteroids potentiate the effects of β_2-agonists on bronchial smooth muscle and prevent and reverse β_2-receptor tachyphylaxis in airways in vitro and in vivo. At a molecular level corticosteroids increase the gene transcription of β_2-receptors in human lung and systemic glucocorti-coids prevent downregulation of β_2-receptors in animal lungs.
Unfortunately inhaled corticosteroids do not appear to prevent the development of tolerance to inhaled β_2-agonists in human airways.

Current use

Systemic corticosteroids

Hydrocortisone is given intravenously in *acute asthma*. While the value of corticosteroids in acute severe asthma has been questioned, others have found that they speed the resolution of attacks. There is no apparent advantage in giving very high doses of intravenous steroids (such as methylprednisolone 1 g). Intravenous steroids are indicated in acute asthma if lung function is less than 30% predicted and in whom there is no significant improvement with nebulized β_2-agonist. Intravenous therapy is usually given until a satisfactory response is obtained and then oral prednisolone may be substituted. Oral prednisolone (40–60 mg) has a similar effect to intravenous hydrocortisone and is easier to administer. Inhaled corticosteroids have no proven effect in acute asthma, but trials with nebulized corticosteroids are underway.

Inhaled corticosteroids

Inhaled corticosteroids have revolutionized the treatment of asthma and are the
most effective anti-asthma drugs
currently available. Inhaled corticosteroids are now recommended as first-
line therapy for all but the mildest of
asthmatic patients. Inhaled corticosteroids should be started in any patient
who needs to use a β-agonist inhaler for
symptom control more than three times
a week. Oral corticosteroids are reserved
for patients who cannot be controlled
on other therapy, the dose being titrated
to the lowest that provides acceptable
control of symptoms. For any patient
taking regular oral corticosteroids objective evidence of corticosteroid responsiveness should be obtained before
maintenance therapy is instituted.

Short courses of oral corticosteroids
(such as 30 mg prednisolone daily for
1–2 weeks) are indicated for exacerbations of asthma, and the dose may be
tailed off over 1 week once the exacerbation is resolved (although the tail-off
period is not strictly necessary, patients
find it reassuring). Nebulized corticosteroids (budesonide 1–2 mg twice
daily) may have a steroid-sparing effect
in more severe asthmatic patients who
are on maintenance oral steroids.

For most patients inhaled corticosteroids should be used twice daily,
which improves compliance, once
control of asthma has been achieved
(which may require four-times daily
dosing initially). If a dose of more than
800 μg daily is used a spacer device
should be used as this reduces the risk
of oropharyngeal side-effects. Inhaled
corticosteroids may be used in children
in the same way as adults and at doses
of 400 μg daily or less there is no
evidence of growth suppression.

Early treatment with inhaled corticosteroids in both adults and children
gives a greater improvement in lung
function than if treatment with inhaled
corticosteroids is delayed (and other
treatments such as bronchodilators are
used) (**Figure 32**). This may reflect the
fact that corticosteroids are able to
modify the underlying inflammatory
process and prevent any structural
changes (fibrosis, smooth muscle
hyperplasia etc.) in the airway as a
result of chronic inflammation. It is not
yet certain how early inhaled corticosteroids should be introduced. There is
evidence for inflammation in the
airways, even when patients have
episodic asthma, but at present it is
recommended that inhaled corticosteroids are introduced when there are

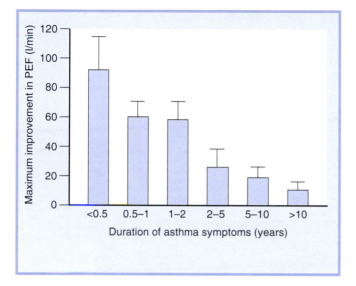

Figure 32
Effect of delaying the introduction of inhaled corticosteroids (from the time of diagnosis of asthma) on the maximum improvement in peak expiratory flow (PEF). (Adapted from Selroos et al (1995))

chronic symptoms (e.g. use of an inhaled β_2-agonist on a daily basis).

Previously it was recommended that inhaled corticosteroids should be introduced in a step-wise manner, increasing the dose until control was achieved. A better approach is to introduce inhaled corticosteroids at a moderate dose (800 µg daily) in all new patients in order to achieve effective control of the inflammation rapidly, and then to decrease the dose once control has been achieved (at least 3 months may be needed for the maximal effects of inhaled cortico-

steroids on airway hyperresponsiveness). Furthermore, there is increasing evidence that it is better to add a long-acting inhaled β_2-agonist, theophylline or anti-leukotriene, than to go to high doses of inhaled corticosteroids in patients not controlled on 800 µg daily of inhaled corticosteroids or more, as this gives better control and there is less risk of systemic side-effects (**Figure 33**).

Corticosteroid resistance

Some patients, usually with severe asthma, apparently fail to respond to

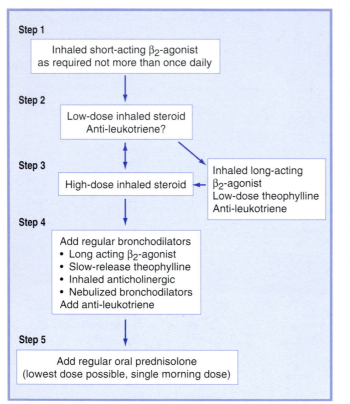

Figure 33
How inhaled corticosteroids fit into asthma treatment guidelines. Inhaled corticosteroids are introduced in any patient who needs to use an inhaled β₂-agonist on a daily basis. It is preferable to start with a moderate dose to achieve rapid control and then to reduce the dose once control is achieved to the minimal dose that maintains control. In patients who are still symptomatic despite 800 µg daily, it is preferable to add a long-acting inhaled β₂-agonist, low-dose theophylline or an anti-leukotriene than increasing inhaled corticosteroids to high doses

corticosteroids. Corticosteroid-resistant asthma is likely to be due to an increase in binding of the glucocorticoid receptor to the transcription factor AP-1, due to increased activation of AP-1.

COPD patients occasionally respond to corticosteroids and these patients are likely to be undiagnosed asthmatics.

Corticosteroids have no objective short-term benefit on airway function in patients with true chronic bronchitis, although they may often produce subjective benefit because of their euphoric effect. There is no convincing evidence that inhaled corticosteroids delay the progressive fall in lung function seen in patients with COPD.

Therapeutic choices

Several highly potent topical cortico-steroids are now available for the treatment of asthma (**Figure 34**).

Beclomethasone dipropionate (BDP), *budesonide* and *fluticasone propionate* (FP) are available for inhaled use in MDI and dry powder formulations.

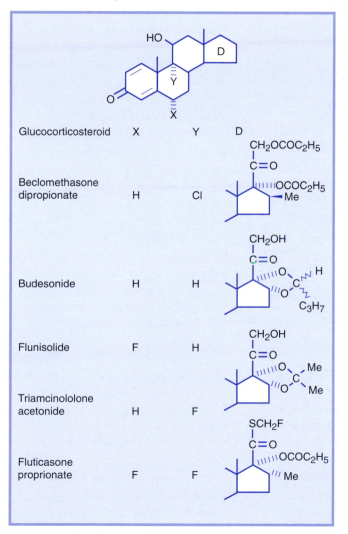

Glucocorticosteroid	X	Y	D
Beclomethasone dipropionate	H	Cl	
Budesonide	H	H	
Flunisolide	F	H	
Triamcinololone acetonide	H	F	
Fluticasone proprionate	F	F	

Figure 34
Structure of inhaled corticosteroids available for asthma therapy

Both inhaled corticosteroids are equally effective as anti-asthma drugs and have a similar potency. At high doses (>1000 µg) budesonide and FP have fewer systemic effects than BDP, and this may be because of increased first pass metabolism of any swallowed budesonide. The type of delivery system is important in the comparison of inhaled corticosteroids. When doses of inhaled corticosteroids exceed 800 µg daily a large volume spacer is recommended as this will reduce any oropharyngeal deposition and hence gastrointestinal absorption, thus reducing any differences between BDP and budesonide. In some countries *flunisolide* and *triamcinolone acetonide* are also available but there is little information available about their systemic absorption and efficacy in asthma.

Nebulized corticosteroids have now been introduced. Nebulized budesonide has been found to be effective in controlling asthma in infants and in adults with severe asthma. It is expensive and may work by giving systemic levels that could be much more cheaply achieved by supplementary oral corticosteroids. Local side-effects include ulceration of the mouth and lips.

Side-effects

Pharmacokinetics

The pharmacokinetics of inhaled corticosteroids are important in relation to systemic effects (**Figure 35**). The fraction of steroid that is inhaled into the lungs acts locally on the airway mucosa and may be absorbed from the airway and alveolar surface and therefore reach the systemic circulation. The fraction of inhaled steroid that is deposited in the oropharynx is swallowed and absorbed from the gut. The absorbed fraction may be metabolized in the liver before reaching the systemic circulation. Budesonide and fluticasone have a greater first pass metabolism than BDP and are less likely to produce systemic effects at high inhaled doses. The use of a large volume spacer chamber reduces oropharyngeal deposition and therefore reduces systemic absorption of corticosteroids. Similarly rinsing the mouth and discarding the rinse has a similar effect and this procedure should be used with high-dose dry powder corticosteroid inhalers, since spacer chambers cannot be used with these devices.

Systemic side-effects

Corticosteroids inhibit adrenocorticotropic hormone (ACTH) and cortisol

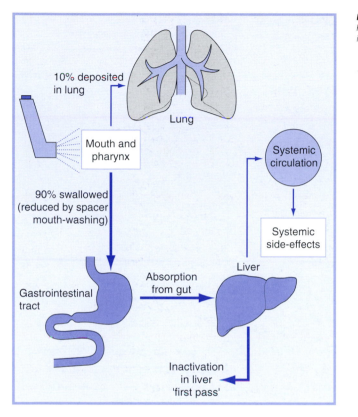

Figure 35
Pharmacokinetics of inhaled steroids

secretion by a negative feedback effect on the pituitary gland. Hypothalamo–pituitary–adrenal (HPA) axis suppression is dependent on dose, and usually only occurs when a dose of prednisolone greater than 7.5–10 mg daily is used. Significant suppression after short courses of corticosteroid therapy is not usually a problem, but prolonged suppression may occur after several months or years. Corticosteroid doses after prolonged oral therapy must therefore be reduced slowly. Symptoms of 'steroid withdrawal syndrome' include lassitude, musculo-skeletal pains and occasionally fever.

HPA suppression with inhaled cortico-steroids is seen only when the daily inhaled dose exceeds 2000 µg daily.

Side-effects of long-term oral cortico-steroid therapy are well described and include fluid retention, increased appetite, weight gain, osteoporosis, capillary fragility, hypertension, peptic ulceration, diabetes, cataracts and psychosis. Their frequency tends to increase with age. Very occasionally adverse reactions (such as anaphylaxis) to intravenous hydrocortisone have been described, particularly in aspirin-sensitive asthmatics.

Corticosteroids have side-effects due to systemic absorption and local side-effects at the sites of deposition in the respiratory tract (**Table 6**). The incidence of systemic side-effects after inhaled corticosteroids is an important consideration. Systemic absorption occurs not only from the gastrointesti-nal tract, but also from the lung, so that all systemic corticosteroids currently available have some systemic absorption. Initial studies suggested that adrenal suppression only occurred when inhaled doses over 1500–2000 µg daily were used. More sensitive measurements of systemic effects include indices of bone metabolism,

Table 6
Side-effects of inhaled corticosteroids

Local side-effects
- Dysphonia
- Oropharyngeal candidiasis
- Cough

Systemic side-effects
- Adrenal suppression
- Growth suppression
- Bruising
- Osteoporosis
- Cataracts
- Glaucoma
- Metabolic abnormalities (glucose, insulin, triglycerides)
- Psychiatric disturbances

such as serum osteocalcin and urinary pyridinium cross-links, and in children knemometry, which may be increased with inhaled doses as low as 800 µg in some patients. The clinical relevance of these measurements is not yet clear however. Nevertheless it is important to reduce the likelihood of systemic effects by using the lowest dose of inhaled corticosteroid needed to control the asthma, by the use of a large volume spacer to reduce oropha-ryngeal deposition (and therefore the fraction absorbed from the gastro-intestinal tract).

Several systemic effects of inhaled corticosteroids have been described and include dermal thinning and skin capillary fragility, which is relatively common in elderly patients after high-dose inhaled corticosteroids. Other side-effects such as cataract formation and osteoporosis are reported, but often in patients who are also receiving courses of oral corticosteroids. There has been particular concern about the use of inhaled corticosteroids in children because of growth suppression. Most studies have been reassuring in that doses of 400 μg or less have not been associated with impaired growth, and there may even be a growth spurt as asthma is better controlled. A meta-analysis of over 20 studies with inhaled BDP showed no effect on growth or overall height of children.

Local side-effects

Inhaled corticosteroids may have *local side-effects* due to the deposition of inhaled corticosteroid in the oropharynx. The most common problem is hoarseness and weakness of the voice (dysphonia) which is due to laryngeal deposition. It may occur in up to 40% of patients and is noticed particularly by patients who need to use their voices during their work (lecturers, teachers and singers). It may be due to atrophy of the vocal cords. Throat irritation and coughing after inhalation are common with MDIs and appear to be due to the additives, since these problems are not usually seen if the patient switches to the dry powder inhalers. Oropharyngeal candidiasis may occur in 5% of patients. The incidence of local side-effects may be related to the local concentrations of corticosteroid deposited and may be reduced by the use of large volume spacers, which markedly reduce oropharyngeal deposition. Local side-effects are also less likely when inhaled corticosteroids are used twice daily rather than four times daily. There is no evidence for atrophy of the lining of the airway, or of an increase in lung infections (including tuberculosis) after inhaled corticosteroids.

Adverse effects of corticosteroids in children

A number of studies in children have shown that inhaled corticosteroids even in reasonable doses can reduce adrenal function as shown by sensitive and appropriate tests such as the measurement of 24-hour urinary free cortisol or frequent monitoring of plasma cortisol. There are differences between drugs and the more modern drugs, such as budesonide or fluticasone, are less likely to have adverse effects as compared with older drugs such as beclomethasone. Although clinically evident adrenal insufficiency has not been a problem in children taking reasonable doses of inhaled corticosteroids provided they have not also been receiving oral corticosteroids, it is wise to keep the dose of inhaled corticosteroid to the lowest that controls symptoms adequately.

While osteoporosis from the use of inhaled corticosteroids has not been reported in children a particular worry in this age group is the possibility of growth suppression. Even normal doses of inhaled corticosteroids can reduce lower leg growth measured by knemometry in a dose-dependent fashion in the short term. The suppression is much less than that seen with oral corticosteroids and the newer inhaled corticosteroids seen to have less of this potentially adverse effect. However, the studies of the effect of inhaled corticosteroids on short-term growth were undertaken in children with very mild asthma so that any positive effect on growth resulting

from the beneficial effect of the inhaled corticosteroid on the asthma would not have been seen. In a long-term study of asthmatic children it has been shown that inadequate control of the asthma but not the use of corticosteroids adversely affects growth. In a very careful study of growth in asthmatic children who were followed until they had passed through puberty the final height of asthmatics was on average just what was predicted by the height centile at entry to the study at a mean age of 7.5 years when there was no evidence of growth retardation. It has also been noted that asthmatic children have on average some delay in the onset of puberty that is unrelated to the type of drug they are receiving and this may appear to make the adolescent asthmatic grow more slowly. Several controlled studies in children with asthma and in adults who had asthma as children have shown that while there may be a small degree of growth impairment with oral therapy there is none with inhaled therapy even with higher doses, longer use or worse asthma.

Further reading

Barnes PJ (1995) Inhaled glucocorticoids for asthma. *New Engl J Med* **332:** 868–75.

Barnes PJ (1996) Mechanism of action of glucocorticoids in asthma. *Am J Respir Crit Care Med* **154:** S21–7.

Barnes PJ, Greening AP and Crompton GK (1995) Glucocorticoid resistance in asthma. *Am J Respir Crit Care Med* **152**(Suppl 6): S125–40.

Barnes PJ, Pedersen S and Busse WW (1998) Efficacy and safety of inhaled corticosteroids: an update. *Am J Respir Crit Care Med* **157:** S1–53.

Efthimou J, Barnes PJ (1998) Effect of inhaled steroids on bone and growth. *Eur Respir J* **11:** 1167–77.

Lipworth BJ (1995) New perspectives in drug delivery and systemic bioactivity. *Thorax* **50:** 105–10.

Selroos O, Pietinalho A, Lofroos AB et al (1995) Effect of early vs late intervention with inhaled corticosteroids in asthma. *Chest* **108:** 1228–34.

Other therapies

4

Several other classes of drug may control the symptoms of asthma and are used in long-term treatment, but do not act as symptom relievers in the same way as short-acting β_2-agonists. While these drugs do not suppress the inflammation of asthma as effectively as corticosteroids, they appear to act on some aspect of the inflammatory process. Thus, antihistamines may be considered anti-inflammatory in that they inhibit the effects of an inflammatory mediator, but they do not suppress the inflammatory process in asthma. Long-acting inhaled β_2-agonists, while classified as bronchodilators, are also used in long-term control of asthma, despite the fact that they do not appear to have any anti-inflammatory action.

Cromones

Cromones include *sodium cromoglycate* and *nedocromil sodium*. Cromoglycate is a derivative of khellin, an Egyptian herbal remedy which was found to protect against allergen challenge without bronchodilator effect. Nedocromil sodium is structurally related and has very similar clinical effects, although there is some evidence that it is more potent.

Mode of action

Initial investigations indicated that cromoglycate inhibited the release of mediators by allergen in passively sensitized human and animal lung, and inhibited passive cutaneous anaphylaxis in rat, although it was without effect in guinea pig. This activity was attributed to stabilization of the mast cell membrane and thus cromoglycate was classified as a mast-cell stabilizer. However, cromoglycate has a rather low potency in stabilizing human lung mast cells, and other drugs that are more potent in this respect have little or no effect in clinical asthma. This has raised doubts about mast-cell stabilization as the major mode of action of cromoglycate.

Cromones potently inhibit bronchoconstriction induced by sulphur dioxide, metabisulphite and bradykinin, which are believed to act through activation of sensory nerves in the airways. In dogs cromones suppress firing of unmyelinated C-fibre nerve endings,

reinforcing the view that it might be acting to suppress sensory nerve activation and thus neurogenic inflammation. Cromones have variable inhibitory actions on other inflammatory cells that may participate in allergic inflammation, including macrophages and eosinophils. In vivo cromoglycate is capable of blocking the early response to allergen (which may be mediated by mast cells) but also the late response and airway hyperresponsiveness, which are more likely to be mediated by macrophage and eosinophil interactions. There is also evidence that long-term treatment with cromones reduces airway hyperresponsiveness.

The molecular mechanism of action of cromones is not understood, but recent evidence suggests that they may block a particular type of chloride channel that may be expressed in sensory nerves, mast cells and other inflammatory cells. It remains to be explained why cromones are only effective in allergic inflammation.

Current use

Cromoglycate is a prophylactic treatment and needs to be given regularly. Cromoglycate protects against various indirect bronchoconstrictor stimuli, such as exercise and fog. It is only effective in mild asthma, but does not appear to be effective in all patients and there seems no sure way of predicting which patients are likely to respond. Cromoglycate is often the anti-inflammatory drug of first choice in children because it has almost no side-effects, although recent controlled trials indicate that it may have little or no effect in young asthmatics. In adults corticosteroids by inhalation are preferred as they are effective in all patients, although adults with mild asthma (even when it is non-allergic in type) do respond to cromoglycate. Cromoglycate has to be given four-times daily to provide good protection, which makes it less useful than inhaled corticosteroids that may be given twice daily. It may also be taken prior to exercise in children with exercise-induced asthma that is not blocked by an inhaled β-agonist. In clinical practice nedocromil has a similar efficacy to cromoglycate and is therefore indicated in patients with mild asthma, but the unpleasant taste makes cromoglycate preferable to many patients. There is an increasing tendency to substitute inhaled corticosteroids for cromogly-cate in adults and children, as cortico-steroids are more effective, more convenient to use (once or twice daily versus four times daily), cheaper and at comparable doses have no side-effects.

Side-effects

Cromoglycate is one of the safest drugs available and side-effects are extremely rare. The dry powder inhaler may cause throat irritation, coughing and, occasion-ally, wheezing but this is usually prevented by prior administration of β_2-agonist inhaler. Very rarely a transient rash and urticaria are seen and a few cases of pulmonary eosinophilia have been reported, all of which are due to hypersensitivity. Side-effects with nedocromil are not usually a problem although some patients have noticed a sensation of flushing after using the inhaler. Many patients find the bitter taste unpleasant, but a menthol-flavoured version is now available which seems to overcome this problem.

Anti-leukotrienes

Anti-leukotrienes are a new class of anti-asthma agent that has recently been introduced into clinical practice.

Mode of action

Elevated levels of these leukotrienes are detected in BAL fluid from

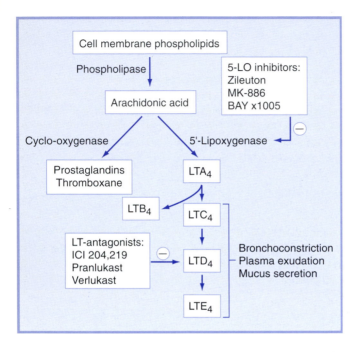

Figure 36
Generation of cysteinyl-leukotrienes from arachidonic acid by 5'-lipoxygenase

asthmatics and elevated LTE_4 levels in the urine of asthmatics. Cysteinyl-leukotrienes (LTC_4, LTD_4, LTE_4) are generated from arachidonic acid by the rate-limiting enzyme 5'-lipoxygenase (5-LO) (**Figure 36**). Cys-leukotrienes are potent constrictors of human airways in vitro and in vivo, cause airway microvascular leakage in animals and stimulate airway mucus secretion (**Figure 37**). These effects are all mediated in human airways via cys-LT_1 receptors. Potent cys-LT_1 antagonists have now been developed and several are now entering the clinic. Inhibitors of the rate-limiting enzyme 5-LO have also been developed. These drugs may be either direct enzyme inhibitors (such as zileuton) or inhibitors of 5'-lipoxygenase activating protein (FLAP) that is necessary for activation of 5'-

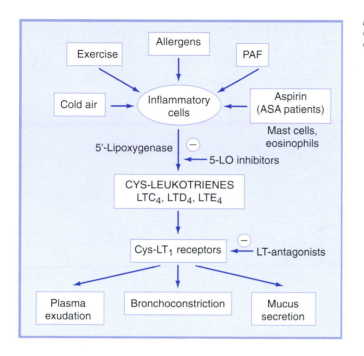

Figure 37
Cellular origin and effects of cysteinyl-leukotrienes

lipoxygenase. The clinical effects of leukotriene antagonists and 5-LO inhibitors are very similar.

Zafirlukast, pranlukast and *montelukast* are potent antagonists that markedly inhibit the bronchoconstrictor response to inhaled leukotrienes. In addition, they reduce allergen-induced responses, exercise and cold-air-induced asthma by approximately 50%, and aspirin-induced responses in aspirin-sensitive asthmatics completely. 5-LO inhibitors are equally effective.

In recent studies anti-leukotrienes have also been demonstrated to have mild anti-inflammatory effects and may reduce eosinophilic inflammation that may be provoked by cysteinyl-leukotrienes.

Clinical use

In clinical studies anti-leukotrienes may have a small bronchodilator effect, indicating that leukotrienes contribute to baseline bronchoconstriction in asthma. Long-term administration reduces asthma symptoms and the need for rescue β_2-agonists and improves lung function parameters. The effects are not as great as expected with inhaled corticosteroids, but few direct comparisons have so far been made in controlled trials. Recent studies suggest that anti-leukotrienes may be useful in patients not

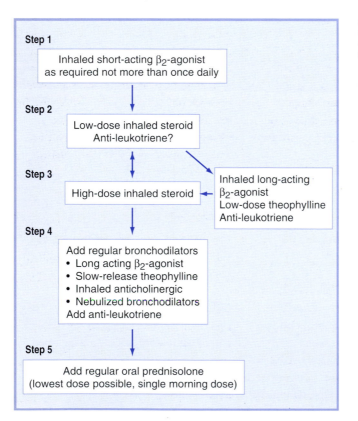

Figure 38
Place of anti-leukotrienes in the asthma treatment guidelines

controlled on inhaled corticosteroids and may be as effective or more effective than doubling the dose of inhaled corticosteroids (as are inhaled long-acting β_2-agonists and theophylline) (**Figure 38**). Corticosteroids are not effective in inhibiting the production of leukotrienes in asthma and therefore anti-leukotrienes may be usefully combined with inhaled corticosteroids, especially in patients with more severe asthma.

There appear to be differences between patients in the magnitude of response to anti-leukotrienes, but so far it is impossible to predict which patients will respond best, apart from the rare patients with aspirin-sensitive asthma.

A major advantage of anti-leukotrienes is that they are orally active and this is likely to make compliance with long-term therapy better than with inhaled drugs. Montelukast is effective as a once daily administration and this may further improve compliance. Their place in asthma management has not yet been established, but they may be indicated in mild asthma as an alternative to inhaled corticosteroids or cromones, or as a supplement to inhaled corticosteroids. However, these treatments are expensive and a trial of therapy may be indicated to determine which patients will benefit most.

Side-effects

Side-effects do not seem to be a problem at present and this may be because leukotrienes are only produced under pathological circumstances. Some drugs produce mild liver dysfunction, so that it is important to do liver functions tests. A few cases of the very rare Churg–Strauss syndrome (systemic vasculitis with eosinophilia and asthma) have been observed with patients on Zafirlukast, but this may be because reduction in oral corticosteroids, made possible by the anti-leukotriene, allows this vasculitis to flare up.

Ketotifen

Ketotifen is described as a prophylactic anti-asthma compound. Its predominant effect is H_1-receptor antagonism and it is this antihistaminic effect that accounts for its sedative effect. Ketotifen has little effect in clinical asthma, either in acute challenge, on airway hyperresponsiveness or on clinical symptoms. A long-term placebo control trial or oral ketotifen in children with mild asthma showed no significant clinical benefit. It is claimed that ketotifen has disease-modifying effects if started early in asthma in children and may even prevent the development of asthma in atopic children. More carefully controlled studies are needed to assess the validity of these claims.

Immunosuppressive/cortico-steroid-sparing therapy

Immunosuppressive therapy has been considered in asthma when other treatments have been unsuccessful and when reduction in the dose of oral corticosteroids is required. They are therefore only indicated in a very small proportion of asthmatic patients at present.

Methotrexate

Low-dose methotrexate (15 mg weekly) has been shown to have a steroid-sparing effect in asthma and may be indicated when oral corticosteroids are contraindicated because of unacceptable side-effects (e.g. in postmenopausal women when osteoporosis is a problem). Some patients show better responses than others, but whether a patient will experience a useful corticosteroid-sparing effect is unpredictable. In some studies no

useful beneficial effect is reported. Side-effects of methotrexate are relatively common and include nausea (reduced if methotrexate is given as a weekly *injection*), blood dyscrasias and hepatic damage. Careful monitoring of such patients (monthly blood counts and liver enzymes) is essential. Methotrexate has been found to be disappointing in most people's clinical experience.

Gold

Gold has long been used in the treatment of chronic arthritis. There is anecdotal evidence that it may also be useful in asthma, and it has been used in Japan for many years. A controlled trial of an oral gold preparation (Auranofin) demonstrated some corticosteroid-sparing effect in chronic asthmatic patients maintained on oral corticosteroids. Side-effects such as skin rashes and nephropathy are a limiting factor.

Cyclosporin A

Cyclosporin A is active against CD4+ lymphocytes and is therefore potentially useful in asthma in which these cells are implicated. A trial of low-dose oral cyclosporin A in patients with corticosteroid-dependent asthma indicated that it can improve control of symptoms in patients with severe asthma on oral corticosteroids, but other trials have been unimpressive. Its use is likely to be limited by severe side-effects, such as nephrotoxicity and hypertension, which are common. In clinical practice it is very disappointing as a corticosteroid-sparing agent.

Intravenous immunoglobulin

Intravenous immunoglobulin has been reported to have corticosteroid-sparing effects in corticosteroid dependent asthma, when high doses were used (2 g/kg), although in a controlled trial in children at lower doses it was ineffective. This is an extremely expensive treatment that cannot on present evidence be recommended.

Treatments that are not effective

Several other treatments have been used in asthma treatment and these include drugs as well as non-pharmacological approaches.

Calcium antagonists

There was considerable interest about 10 years ago in the possibility that calcium antagonists may be useful as bronchodilators in asthma, but studies with nifedipine, verapamil, diltiazem and other voltage-dependent calcium antagonists showed only minor protective effects in airway challenge studies and no significant bronchodilator effects. There is no evidence that these drugs have any useful effect in clinical asthma.

Antihistamines

Non-sedative antihistamines, such as *terfenadine* annd *loratadine*, have proved useful in the control of allergic rhinitis, but are not effective in the control of clinical asthma, despite the fact that they are able to reduce the bronchoconstrictor response to allergen in challenge studies. It is likely that conventional doses of antihistamines are too low. New antihistamines, such as cetirizine and azelastine have a small beneficial effect on asthma control and may be acting via a mechanism unrelated to H_1-receptor antagonism.

α-Adrenoreceptor antagonists

α-Receptor blockers were tried out in asthma in the light of evidence for bronchoconstrictor α-receptors in asthmatic airways in vitro. More recent studies have questioned the existence of α-receptors that mediate bronchoconstriction in asthma, however. Phentolamine and indoramin were shown to have some protective effect in certain asthma challenges, but have other pharmacological actions that could explain their efficacy. A more specific α-antagonist such as prazosin was without significant bronchodilator or protective effect, and α-receptor antagonists have not proved useful in the clinical management of asthma.

Mucolytics

Mucus plugging is a predominant feature of asthma and mucus glycoproteins are an important constituent of these plugs. There is often also marked goblet cell hyperplasia in asthmatic airways. This has suggested that agents that reduce viscosity may be useful in the management of chronic (particularly severe) asthma. In practice mucolytic drugs, such as oral carbocysteine, methylcysteine, N-acetylcysteine and bromhexine are well tolerated, and whilst they are capable of reducing sputum viscosity in vitro, they do not appear to have any useful clinical effect in asthma or in COPD.

Immunotherapy

Although desensitizing injections to grass pollen and house-dust mite have some efficacy in allergic rhinitis, there is little evidence for significant efficacy in asthma, and the high incidence of local side-effects and the risk of anaphylaxis argue against this therapy when safe and more effective alternatives are available. A recent controlled trials showed that immunotherapy with mixed allergens in children was ineffective for asthma control. However, there are important advances in the development of safer and more effective allergen preparations, using purified or recombinant allergens (e.g. *DerP1*) or peptide fragments that preserve allergenicity.

Allergen avoidance

The house-dust mite allergen *DerP1* is the most potent allergen in terms of sensitization and persistence of asthma and is the most common indoor allergen. There is persuasive epidemiological evidence that the level of exposure to house-dust mite is an important determinant of asthma severity and the level of airway hyperresponsiveness. Indeed the increasing tendency in temperate climates to live in 'tight' houses, with increased humidity in bedrooms, together with the tendency to carpet bedrooms may be one of the factors contributing to the increased prevalence of asthma. Avoidance of allergens in the home (especially house-dust mite and cat) is an important part of the treatment strategy, although effective avoidance is very complicated and it is difficult to achieve and maintain avoidance. Getting rid of carpets and curtains in the bedroom, covering the mattress with plastic and increasing ventilation are the most important measures that have been shown to reduce (but not eradicate) *DerP1*. More intensive treatment involves the use of *acaricide* sprays to kill mites, but these are not that effective and this approach has not convincingly been shown to improve asthma control.

Alternative therapies

Various other non-pharmacological treatments have been advocated for asthma, including acupuncture, homeopathy, yoga, the use of ionizers and various herbal and dietary remedies. Although there may be isolated reports of marginal benefit, most controlled studies have not demonstrated any objective benefit. These therapies may be helpful to the asthmatic patients, however, and may be used provided that the patient continues to take his or her conventional therapy.

Further reading

Barnes PJ (1996) Immunotherapy for asthma: is it worth it? *New Engl J Med* **334:** 531–2.

Barnes PJ, Holgate ST, Laitinen LA and Pauwels R (1995) Asthma mechanisms, determinants of severity and treatment: the role of nedocromil sodium. *Clin Exp Allergy* **25:** 771–87.

Hill SJ and Tattersfield AE (1995) Corticosteroid sparing agents in asthma. *Thorax* **50:** 577–82.

Hoag JE and McFadden ER (1991) Long-term effect of cromolyn sodium on nonspecific bronchial hyperresponsiveness: a review. *Ann Allergy* **66:** 53–63.

Lewith GT and Watkins AJ (1996) Unconventional therapies in asthma: an overview. *Allergy* **51:** 761–9.

O'Byrne PM, Israel E and Drazen JM (1997) Antileukotrienes in the treatment of asthma. *Ann Int Med* **127:** 472–80.

Inhaler devices

5

Asthma is a disease of the bronchial tree in which the airways are narrowed – the result of a combination of bronchospasm, inflammatory infiltration and secretion into the lumen. The most obvious and direct route for delivering drugs to the asthmatic airway is by inhalation and fortunately, most of the medications needed to treat asthma can be delivered by this route. In some cases the choice of inhalation is because the drugs, for example cromones, are without effect when given systematically. In most cases, however, they are given by inhalation because of either speed of onset of action, as with β_2-agonists, or to avoid systemic side-effects, as with corticosteroids. There are now a wide variety of devices on the market for delivering drugs by inhalation and they fall into four broad categories.

Pressurized metered-dose inhaler (pMDI)

The pMDI consists of a reservoir canister containing medication mixed with a chlorofluorocarbon (CFC)

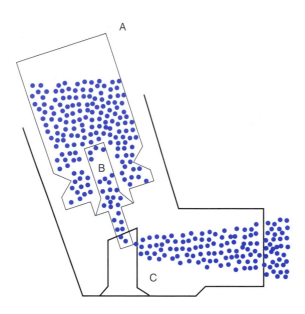

Figure 39
Generic type of pressurized metered-dose inhaler (pMDI) – components described in the text

propellant (currently being replaced by a hydrofluorocarbon (HFC), and a lubricating surfactant. The mixture is released through a metering chamber when the device is activated and a controlled dose is emitted as a spray. The general form of a pMDI is shown in **Figure 39**. The drug is stored under pressure in a metal canister (A) and released through a valve (B) that delivers a fixed dose when the canister is pressed into its mount in the body. The spray is delivered to the mouth piece (C) to be inhaled by the patient.

Pressurized metered-dose inhaler with spacer (pMDI-SP)

Because many patients are unable to co-ordinate well enough to use an MDI correctly, various holding chambers (spacers) have been developed; these are placed between the MDI and the patient. The drug is inhaled from the chamber and co-ordination with the firing of the MDI is no longer important. Most spacers have some type of non-rebreathing valve. Some are large volume, some are much smaller, and

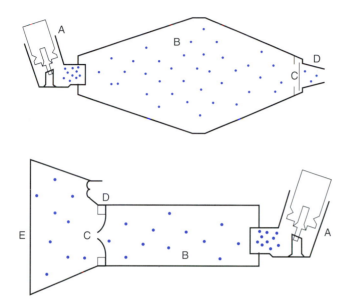

Figure 40a
Generic type of pressurized
metered-dose inhaler and
large volume spacer (pMDI-
SP) suitable for an adult –
schematic representation of
Volumatic and Nebuhaler
spacers – components
described in the text

Figure 40b
Generic type of pressurized
metered-dose inhaler and
small volume spacer with
face mask (pMDI-SP) suitable
for an infant – schematic
representation of
Aerochamber and Babyhaler
spacers – components
described in the text

there are spacers with face masks suitable for infants. The general form of a large volume pMDI-SP suitable for an adult is shown in **Figure 40a**. The drug is discharged from the pMDI (A) into the large volume plastic chamber (B) and inhaled by the patient through a one-way valve (C) via a mouth piece (D). The general form of a small volume pMDI-SP suitable for small children is shown in **Figure 40b**. The drug is discharged from the pMDI (A) into the small volume plastic chamber (B) and inhaled by the patient through a one-way inspiratory valve (C) with expired air passing through a one-way expiratory valve (D) using a face mask (E) covering the mouth and nose.

Dry powder inhaler (DPI)

For many years devices have been available for the delivery of dry powders of medications diluted with suitable inert compounds. These do not contain CFCs and since they are only activated by the inspiratory effort of the patient do not require co-ordination between firing and

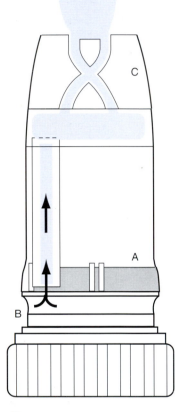

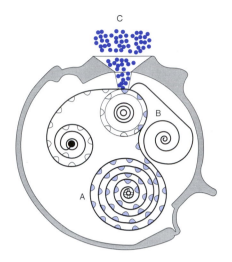

Figure 41b
*Dry powder inhaler (DPI) with blisters of drug –
schematic representation of Accuhaler and Diskus
inhalers – components described in the text*

Figure 41a
*Dry powder inhaler (DPI) with drug reservoir – schematic
representation of Turbohaler inhaler – components
described in the text*

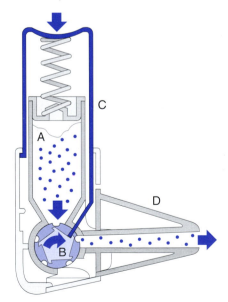

Figure 41c
*Dry powder inhaler (DPI) with drug reservoir resembling a
pMDI – schematic representation of Easyhaler inhaler –
components described in the text*

inspiration as is the case with the pMDI. Initially these delivered single doses of drug are contained in a capsule inserted into the device. More recently various types of multiple dose DPIs have been developed in which the powder is stored within the device. There are three general forms which such devices take. In one type (**Figure 41a**) the drug is stored in a reservoir (A) and a metered dose of powder is scooped out by rotating the base. Inspired air (B) carries the powder to the mouth piece (C) where it is further broken up. In the blister pack type of device (**Figure 41b**) the powder is contained in small blisters attached to a strip (A) the backing of which is peeled off (B) so that the drug is dispersed through the mouth piece (C) by the inspired air. A novel type of DPI which resembles a pMDI in shape is shown in **Figure 41c**. In this device the powder is held in a plastic canister (A) from which a metering device (B) liberates a fixed amount when the spring-loaded plunger (C) is pressed into the mount. Inspired air then entrains the particles of drug which are inhaled through the mouth piece (D).

Jet nebulizer (NEB)

The oldest type of inhalation devices delivered the drug by nebulizing the medication to produce a cloud of medication. In its modern form this is accomplished by passing a jet of air from a compressor over a solution of the drug contained in a reservoir. Some types of NEB operate continuously and some are triggered by the patient. The general form of this type of device is shown in **Figure 42a**. The jet of air from the compressor (A) entrains some of the liquid drug from the reservoir (B) which is broken into small particles as it hits a baffle (C) and is then delivered as a mist to the patient who inhales it either from an open mask or from a mouth piece (D).

Ultrasonic nebulizer (US-NEB)

A less common type of nebulizer for use by asthmatics is the ultrasonic nebulizer which produces a cloud of dug by having a plate which vibrates at very high frequency in contact with the drug reservoir. The general form of this type of device is shown in **Figure 42b**. A piezoelectric crystal is made to vibrate by an electric current (A) and this produces a spray above the liquid drug contained in the reservoir (B). The drug particles are separated by impinging on a baffle (C) and delivered to the patient continuously or intermittently through a mouth piece (D) with

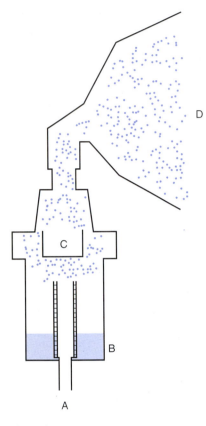

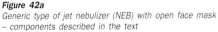

Figure 42a
Generic type of jet nebulizer (NEB) with open face mask – components described in the text

Figure 42b
Generic type of ultrasonic nebulizer (US-NEB) with mouth piece and one-way valves – components described in the text

one-way valves in a similar fashion to the regular jet type of NEB.

Whatever type of inhalation device is used its efficacy depends upon the

characteristics of the particles it produces which reach the patient and the ability of the patient to use the device correctly. In many instances the drug can theoretically be delivered equally well by different types of devices but the ability of the patient to use the device may impose severe restrictions on the type that can be used efficiently. Because of the complex factors involved, it is often impossible to know exactly how much drug is reaching the patient from a given device and how far the drug penetrates into the airways. This makes comparisons of different devices very difficult and often impossible. Under these circumstances clinical trials are used to determine the efficacy of a particular system in controlling symptoms or altering lung function while attention is paid to the side-effects of the undesirable systemic absorption of the drug.

The importance of particle size

Only certain particles can reach the lungs when inhaled because if they are too large they impact on the apparatus or in the mouth and pharynx and if they are too small they may never come to rest in the lungs and are simply breathed out. All therapeutic agents for inhalation are aerosols of either liquid or solid particles dispersed in a gas with a particle size range in the aerosol designed to ensure deposition in the lung. The efficacy of the

aerosol depends not only upon the size distribution of the particles but also on the mass of drug contained in particles of a size likely to reach the target. The behaviour of the particles in an aerosol also depends on their shape and for the purposes of studying their behaviour this is defined in terms of their aerodynamic diameter that is the diameter of a sphere of water which would fall in still air with the same final velocity as the irregular shaped particle under consideration. The distribution of the particles according to their aerodynamic diameter and either number or size defines the aerosol. The most useful parameter describing this distribution is the mass median aerodynamic diameter (MMAD). This is the size of the particle such that half the mass of the aerosol is contained in particles that are larger and half in particles that are smaller. The most useful MMAD for therapeutic aerosols is between 1 and 6 μm since particles smaller than 1 μm behave like a gas and are breathed out while those larger than 6 μm may never reach the airways. Within the airways the deposition of particles occurs by impaction, sedimentation and diffusion and particles of different sizes will deposit predominantly in different regions. Thus particles of about 5 μm or larger in size will deposit mainly on the airway surface and less in the peripheral lung tissue while for particles of about 3 μm, the opposite is true.

Other factors influence the amount and site of deposition of aerosols within the lungs. When airway calibre is reduced or inspiratory flow is increased deposition shifts towards the more proximal airways. This also occurs in healthy children because of the configuration of their airways. Many aerosols are hygroscopic and the particles grow in size when they reach the humid airways resulting in more proximal deposition. When delivered into a humidified respiratory circuit this may result in much of the drug being deposited in the tubing of the apparatus and not reaching the patient at all. During the operation of a jet nebulizer there is a progressive increase in concentration and cooling of drug in the reservoir which results in an increase in droplet size and reduction in output. These effects can be reduced by having a larger volume of solution in the reservoir. The aerosol generated from a pMDI depends upon the design of the apparatus and the vapour pressure of the propellant in the canister. Most pMDIs produce particles of about 3-6 μm MMAD. Because

it is released from the inhaler at a high velocity much of the aerosol impacts in the oropharynx of the patient and the cold jet may be quite unpleasant and cause the patient to cough. Such factors as the volume of the spacer, the presence and stiffness of any valves and the materials used in the construction considerably affect the composition and deposition of the aerosol in metered-dose inhalers with a spacer (pMDI-SP). The overall effect of modern, practical spacers is to produce a finer, slower moving aerosol with less impaction in the oropharynx and greater deposition in the lung. The build up of an electrostatic charge in a spacer also reduces output and this can be avoided by using a metal spacer or by allowing the drug to coat the walls of the spacer by priming it before use. With dry powder inhalers the aerosol comprises the drug diluted with an inert carrier powder and the particle size depends upon the physical characteristics of the device and the speed of inspiration which breaks up the powder on the baffles. Because lactose carrier particles are usually quite large most impact in the oropharynx while the smaller drug particles enter the airway. It is generally believed that a DPI is more efficient at delivering drug to the lungs than a pMDI but probably about as efficient as a pMDI-SP combination.

The site of deposition of the aerosol is important not only because of the desired effect on the airways but also because of potential side-effects due to absorption of the drug, especially when using inhaled corticosteroids. Drug deposited in the lung produces the desired effect on the airway but is also absorbed directly into the systemic circulation without passing through the liver. Drug deposited in the mouth and oropharynx is also absorbed directly into the systemic circulation while drug that is swallowed passes through the liver where it can be rendered harmless. This subject is very complicated because in theory an effective inhaler which delivers a large dose of drug to the airway could also deliver a large dose to the systemic circulation. There are many possible combinations between the site of drug deposition, systemic absorption and first pass metabolism in the liver. Comparisons of different drug delivery systems are difficult but it appears that the use of a pMDI-SP combination improves the therapeutic ratio, that is there is less systemic absorption for a given effect on the airway. Although systemic absorption using a DPI can be high they are also relatively efficient and hence have a similar therapeutic ratio to the pMDI-SP combination.

The importance of inhalation technique

The amount of drug reaching the lungs and the amount deposited in the mouth and oropharynx depends not only on the type of inhaler device but also on the way it is used by the patient. The incorrect use of a pMDI such as firing the device very late in inspiration can result in virtually all of the drug being deposited in the mouth and none in the lungs. Using a pMDI-SP spacer of large volume with stiff valves can result in an infant receiving none of the medication and likewise the use of a DPI by a patient with a very low inspiratory flow rate can greatly reduce the amount of drug entering the lungs. Even nebulizers can be problematic if the patient fails to use them correctly and some infants are quite terrified by the noise of the device and simply refuse to use them. The individual manufacturers recommend the best inhalation technique for their device and this should be explained to the patient by the person prescribing the device. There are certain general principles which apply to the use of the different types of device and each group has its advantages and disadvantages.

Pressurized metered-dose inhaler

The device should be shaken immediately before use and held in an upright position, that is with the reservoir pointing upwards. It should not be inverted or held with the reservoir horizontal. The patient should breathe out, close lips around the mouth piece and then fire the device at the start of a slow, deep inspiration to total lung capacity. The breath should then be held for about 10 seconds before breathing out. Only one dose should be inhaled at a time and under no circumstances should the device be fired more than once during the same inspiration. There is some theoretical advantage to firing the device a little way in front of the widely open mouth but this technique is very prone to mistakes and should not be used under normal circumstances.

The advantages of the pMDI inhalers include the following:

* Devices are small and easily portable

* Generally cheap
* Quick to use.

The disadvantages of the pMDI inhalers include the following:

* Good technique is essential
* Unsuitable for children less than 5-6 years of age
* Unsuitable for elderly, arthritic or patients with coordination problems
* Unsuitable for patients with limited ability to understand their use.

Pressurized metered-dose inhaler with spacer

The pMDI to be used with the spacer should be shaken immediately before use and fixed upright in the appropriate aperture in the spacer. If used with a mouth piece the lips should be kept firmly placed around it to prevent any leak and if used with a face mask the mask should be held firmly over the nose and mouth so that there is no leak of air around the mask. The patient should continue to breathe reasonably deeply and forcibly without pausing from the spacer while the pMDI is fired. About 1-2 deep breaths are usually sufficient after firing for adults and about 3-4 for children. It is essential to be sure that the valves of the spacer are moving correctly – an audible click should be heard with the rigid plastic type and the parents should try to observe the flexible valve movement in those for infants. Some recommend priming the spacer with a few doses to coat the inside and reduce static loss of drug before using the spacer for the first time and not washing it too often. When the treatment calls for two or more doses of medication, it is important that each dose be taken separately; it is not recommended that the pMDI is activated more than once per inspiration or that the spacer is loaded with several doses. When using a pMDI-SP with a face mask to administer corticosteroids to an infant or young child it is recommended that the face be washed afterwards to reduce exposure of the skin around the mouth to the drug.

The advantages of the pMDI-SP inhalers include the following:

- Co-ordination unimportant
- Can be used by patients of all ages
- May reduce systemic absorption
- Relatively inexpensive.

The disadvantages of the pMDI-SP inhalers include the following:

- Devices are bulky and inconvenient
- Valves sometimes stick or become incompetent
- Some infants struggle against the mask and a good seal may not be obtained.

Dry powder inhaler

There are several different types of DPI and it is important to follow the instructions for priming the device as recommended by the manufacturer. One type (Turbohaler) should be held vertically while rotating the base to load the dose while another (Accuhaler, Diskus) requires two levers to be operated to load the dose and open the mouth piece. Another device (Easyhaler) resembles a pMDI in shape and is primed by pressing down the reservoir which makes it easy for the patient to understand if they have previously used a pMDI but they must realize that the drug is not released from the device until they inspire. With all types of DPI the patients should breathe out before closing the lips firmly around the mouth piece. The patient should then inspire as rapidly and deeply as possible. All DPIs are flow dependent and operate best with an inspiratory flow rate of about 60 l/min although some may still be effective at half this rate of inspiration. As with a pMDI the inspiration should be followed by a short breath hold. When taking corticosteroids from a DPI it is recommended that the mouth be washed out afterwards to reduce buccal absorption of the drug.

The advantages of the DPI inhalers include the following:

- Co-ordination between priming and inspiring unimportant
- Can be used for most ages including children from about 5-6 years
- Devices are small and portable.

The disadvantages of the DPI inhalers include the following:

- Require rapid inspiration
- Not suitable for children below the age of 5 years
- Unsuitable for patients with limited ability to understand their use
- Relatively expensive.

Jet nebulizer

The nebulizer should be set up according to the manufacturer's instructions and the appropriate amount of drug diluted with saline if necessary should be placed in the reservoir. It is common practice to use a 2 ml fill because the time of nebulization is reduced to about 6-8 minutes in most devices but there are theoretical advantages in terms of drug delivery to using a larger volume of about 4 ml even though this may take a little longer. Most NEB reservoirs must be held in a vertical position so that the drug does not spill over into the exit from the nebulization chamber. This can easily occur if the device is used for a child who is asleep in bed. The patient should breathe normally from the mouth piece or face mask while the compressor (or ultrasonic device) is run continuously until a cloud of drug is no longer apparent at the exit of the device. If for some reason the patient stops breathing from the NEB it should be turned off until breathing is resumed.

The advantages of the NEB inhalers include the following:

- Co-ordination unimportant
- Can be used for all ages.

The disadvantages of the NEB inhalers include the following:

- Cumbersome equipment
- Requires source of electricity
- Expensive
- Noisy
- Treatment takes a long time
- Disliked by some infants, loathed by others.

Performance of different devices and patient compatibility

Naturally, every manufacturer believes that their device is the best for delivering a drug by inhalation to the patient but unfortunately it is very difficult and in many cases impossible to make accurate comparisons between devices because of the multitude of factors involved. Almost all devices marketed produce particles of respirable size in the 1-6 μm range and rather surprisingly the proportion of the nominal dose released from the device which reaches the lungs is also about 10-20% for the different types of device. For two devices, the Turbohaler and Easyhaler this lung dose may be a bit more (20-30%) and it is usually recommended that the dose of drug delivered by a DPI be reduced somewhat in relation to the same drug delivered from a pMDI alone. Side-effects from systemic absorption especially of corticosteroids depend on the total dose entering the patient and on metabolism in the liver. Systemic absorption is generally less when a pMDI is used with a spacer, presumably because large unwanted particles never reach the patient. The overall clinical efficacy and potential side-effects seem to be very similar for the various DPIs and pMDIs when combined with a spacer.

Given the various advantages and disadvantages of the different devices discussed earlier it is possible to make some general recommendations as to the most suitable type of inhalation device for different types of patients.

Infants and children up to about 5 years of age
• pMDI-SP
• NEB

Children 5-9 years
• pMDI alone – sometimes for technically competent children
• pMDI-SP
• DPI
• NEB – usually only needed for acute exacerabation

Competent older children/adults
• MDI alone
• MDI-SP – recommended for high-dose inhaled corticosteroids
• DPI
• NEB – usually only needed for acute exacerbation

Incompetent older children/adults
• MDI-SP
• DPI – some may be able to use these devices but this must be verified

- NEB – may be needed for cortico-steroids as well as bronchodilators

Further reading

Dolovich MB (1997) Aerosols. In: PJ Barnes, MM Grunstein, AR Leff and AJ Woolcock, eds, *Asthma*. Philadelphia: Lippincott–Raven Publishers.

Pauwels R, Newman S and Borgstrom L (1997) Airway deposition and airway effects of antiasthma drugs delivered from metered-dose inhalers. *Eur Respir J* **10:** 2127–38.

Pedersen S (1996) Inhalers and nebulizers: which to choose and why. *Respir Med* **90:** 69–77.

Asthma management

6

Over the past few years there has been an increase
in the understanding of the pathophysiology of
asthma and the various ways in which the quality of
life of the asthmatic can be improved by successful
management. This has led to the formulation of
guidelines for the management of asthma with a
remarkable degree of international agreement,
although there are small differences based on
national preferences. The guidelines make recommendations for the management of chronic asthma
and for acute exacerbations and take account of
differences between children and adults although
these are now quite minor. They also emphasize the
importance of making the correct diagnosis in the
first place, the evaluation of the severity of the
asthma, providing the patient with the means and
information to be a full partner in management and
the avoidance of undesirable side-effects of treatment.

The diagnosis of asthma

The diagnosis of asthma is based on typical history and clinical findings and backed in some cases by laboratory investigations. In many patients, especially children, cough rather than overt wheezing is a common feature of asthma and this may result in the correct diagnosis being missed. Except for the most severe and poorly treated patients, asthma is a disease in which there is marked variation in the severity of the airways obstruction from time to time often with intervals of apparent complete recovery. There is also marked diurnal variation with symptoms usually being worse at night or early in the morning. Other forms of COPD rarely if ever show this degree of variability.

The correct diagnosis is usually made by taking a careful history, physical examination which may not be helpful between attacks, the judicious use of tests of lung function and the exclusion of other diagnoses by appropriate investigations where relevant. In most patients the diagnosis can be confirmed by a simple test of lung function such as spirometry that shows an obstructive pattern which is improved by the inhalation of a bronchodilator. In some cases the improvement in the forced expired volume in one second (FEV_1) is less than the 15% that is generally accepted as indicating asthma and improvement only occurs after more prolonged treatment usually with a course of corticosteroids.

Airway responsiveness testing

Airway hyperresponsiveness is a cardinal physiological feature of asthma. Tests of bronchial reactivity supplemented by simple tests of lung function can be of major importance in making the diagnosis when it is not clear on clinical grounds. There are various ways of measuring non-specific (i.e. non-allergic) bronchial reactivity of which the simplest is by physical exercise. A fall in FEV_1 of more than 10–15% after 6–8 minutes of hard exercise in a relatively dry climate can be expected in about 70% or more asthmatics but not all patients are capable of this type of exercise challenge. The inhalation of non-isotonic fog or isocapnic hyperventilation mimic exercise-induced asthma to some degree but requires complicated equipment and a considerable degree of patient understanding and co-operation. Bronchial provocation by the inhalation of bronchoconstrictors is performed using either methacholine or histamine as the challenge. More recently the inhalation of AMP has been used since it appears to be a highly sensitive and specific challenge for asthma. The simplest method of performing a challenge is the tidal breathing method in which the agent is nebulized using a simple jet-type nebulizer for 2 minutes. Lung function is measured for 3 minutes after each inhalation and the end point of the test (PC_{20}) is the concentration reached when there has been a 20% fall in FEV_1 from the baseline. In children too young to perform lung function tests the methacholine or adenosine can be delivered to an open face mask and the end point of the challenge can be judged by the appearance of wheezing heard with a stethoscope, mild desaturation determined by pulse oximetry, tachycardia or tachypnoea. Asthmatics generally respond abnormally to both exercise and methacholine challenges while those with other types of chronic lung disease often respond abnormally to methacholine but not to exercise or AMP inhalation. This may be helpful in the differential diagnosis of the patient with chronic airways obstruction. Newer techniques for investigating asthma such as the measurement of nitric oxide levels in exhaled air may prove to be useful in estimating the overall level of airway inflammation but have yet to be fully evaluated.

The differential diagnosis of asthma

In patients with unrelenting symptoms alternative diagnoses should be considered which include:

- *Upper airways disease*: especially in infants and young children.
- *Vocal cord dysfunction*: which typically affects adolescents or young adults and is usually misdiagnosed as asthma. The condition is due to an emotional disorder (probably hysterical) in which there is vocal cord adduction during inspiration and/or expiration. Unlike asthma, symptoms are not worse at night or while asleep and there is no arterial desaturation during an 'attack'.
- *Congenital airway anomalies*: such as tracheomalacia, bronchomalacia and vascular rings.
- *Aspiration*: gastro-oesophageal reflux (GOR) may be associated with asthma in some patients and may be the cause of recurrent airways obstruction even without true asthma.

- *Foreign body aspiration*: most common in 1–3-year-old toddlers. Unilateral wheezing should always raise the suspicion of foreign body aspiration.
- *Tumours*: causing airway obstruction and central airway noisy breathing which may be mistaken for asthma are rare.
- *COPD*: due to chronic bronchitis or emphysema or a combination and most often found in patients who are heavy cigarette smokers. The airways obstruction shows only a minor degree of variability although the differentiation from asthma can be difficult in some patients who may have features of both diseases.
- *Interstitial lung diseases*: may cause chronic breathlessness and hypoxia but are easily distinguished clinically, radiologically and physiologically from asthma although there may be an obstructive component in sarcoidosis.
- *Cardiac disease*: which results in pulmonary oedema or raised pulmonary capillary pressure may cause an obstructive type of lung disease which can certainly be episodic and with symptom-free intervals. The differential diagnosis from asthma should be apparent clinically and by investigation but may be difficult in infancy.
- *Acute viral bronchiolitis*: very common in early infancy occurring in epidemics in the winter and mostly due to infection with the respiratory syncytial virus.
- *Chronic post-bronchiolitic wheezing*: affects up to 40% of infants following acute viral bronchiolitis. The infants have repeated episodes of wheezing which tend to become less severe and less frequent with time and cease after 2–3 years of age.
- *Bronchiolitis obliterans*: an uncommon form of COPD with fixed airways obstruction and persistent wheezing which mostly follow a severe viral infection, but also occur after lung transplantation.
- *Bronchopulmonary dysplasia (BPD)*: a form of generalized chronic obstructive pulmonary disease affecting mainly premature infants who have required intensive care with mechanical ventilation and high levels of inspired oxygen.
- *Primary ciliary dyskinesia*: the 'immotile cilia syndrome' affects a small proportion of children who suffer repeated respiratory infections, otitis media and sinusitis but may present with a relatively mild

form of chronic obstructive pulmonary disease that is often mistaken for asthma or cystic fibrosis. Some patients only present in adult life and some are found during the investigation of male infertility which is a feature of the disease.

- *Cystic fibrosis (CF)*: an autosomal recessive disorder which in most patients causes severe and progressive lung disease and pancreatic insufficiency and results in bronchiectasis. In milder genetic variants the patient may only present in adult life and again may be found during the investigation of male infertility which is also a feature of CF.
- *Alpha-1 anti-trypsin deficiency*: is a rare autosomal recessive inborn error of defence against damage by inflammation, especially that induced by cigarette smoking, which leads to a severe and generalized form of emphysema. The lung disease is extremely rare in infancy and childhood and normally only appears in early or middle adult life.

The differentiation of these conditions from asthma depends on the proper use of appropriate investigations to supplement the clinical data. In adults many patients with COPD are misdiagnosed as having asthma and vice versa, while in children, many with congenital airway anomalies are usually thought initially to have asthma. Vocal cord dysfunction is particularly problematic and many patients with this condition receive large amounts of medication for asthma and not infrequently get admitted to intensive care units. The differential diagnosis in the wheezy infant is very problematical and the differentiation between asthma and post-bronchiolitic wheezing may be impossible.

Classification of asthma severity

Once the diagnosis of asthma has been made the decision as to the best management to recommend for the patient depends on an evaluation of the severity of the condition. The nature of the attacks of asthma and the pattern of recurrence varies considerably from patient to patient and this has an important bearing on treatment. In order to develop a rational approach to management it is necessary to have a reasonable and practical method of classification. The various guidelines prepared to help with asthma management attempt to provide a classification of asthma severity. This may be described in terms of the overall amount of disturbance the disease causes the patient and the family without being unduly influenced by the severity of the individual attack of asthma. The amount of disturbance can be evaluated as follows:

• The number of daytime attacks lasting more than 24 hours and needing extra medication
• The presence of completely symptom-free intervals lasting more than 4 weeks without medication
• The frequency of waking at night because of asthma symptoms
• The amount of absence from work or school because of asthma
• The ability of the patient to undertake a normal amount of physical activity
• The number and type of medications required on a regular daily basis
• The frequency of using extra relief medications on an 'as needed' basis
• The frequency of visits to the doctor or Emergency Room
• The frequency of hospital admissions for moderate to severe exacerbations

• The frequency of any life-threatening episodes of acute asthma requiring intensive care.

Based on this type of data averaged over the previous year or two the asthma severity may be classified in one of the following ways which mostly relate to the patient who has not yet been established on optimal treatment.

Mild Asthma: Discrete attacks for no more than 1–2 days occurring no more often than once per month with symptom free intervals or very brief attacks occurring no more than twice per week. Attacks respond readily to β_2-agonist therapy and do not cause the patient to miss more than the occasional day of work or schooling.

Moderate Asthma: Attacks more often than twice weekly with occasional more prolonged exacerbations and requiring frequent or daily medication for relief of symptoms. Such patients may well miss occasional days of work or schooling without adequate treatment.

Severe Asthma: Continuous or virtually continuous symptoms with occasional prolonged severe exacerbations and requiring daily medication for relief of symptoms which only respond adequately to corticosteroids. Such patients often suffer from a reduction in their quality of life, miss some work or schooling and are normally unable to keep pace with their peers without adequate treatment.

Mild and moderate asthma may well be seasonal with complete or virtually complete freedom from symptoms once the relevant season (often spring or winter) is over. Severe asthma is rarely seasonal although the severity of symptoms (and need for treatment) may fluctuate from time to time. There are two other forms of asthma which do not fit readily into the above classification and are seen from time to time.

Sudden life-threatening asthma

A few asthmatics suffer from infrequent but devastatingly severe attacks of asthma. Often the onset of an attack is unpredictable although this form of asthma may occur in patients with marked specific allergy especially food allergy. The attack may necessitate admission to an intensive care unit and ventilatory support but it is not uncommon for the patient to be totally symptom-free in the intervals between attacks. They represent a very high-risk group and their management is problematical.

Whatever the overall pattern of asthma as described above the severity of the individual attack varies from time to time even in the same patient. It is important to note that there is no direct link between the overall severity of the asthma and the severity of the attacks. It is true that most patients with mild asthma suffer from mild attacks but it is not at all rare for such a patient to have a moderate or severe attack from time to time and this does not alter the fact that the pattern of attack frequency is still mild. At the other end of the scale, most patients with severe asthma have mild or moderate attacks that are nevertheless so frequent as to disturb their everyday activities and only rarely are the attacks both frequent and severe. The following classification represents a summary of the various definitions of attack severity that have been proposed.

Mild/moderate non-life-threatening attack:
- Wheezing or coughing without severe distress
- Able to talk normally
- Little or no tachypnoea

- No desaturation (if measured)
- Peak flow >50% predicted (if measured)
- Excellent response to β_2-agonist therapy.

Moderate/severe non-life-threatening attack:
- Wheezing or coughing with moderate distress
- Unable to talk normally, speaks in phrases
- Moderate tachypnoea and tachycardia
- Saturation 90–95% (if measured)
- Peak flow <50% predicted (if measured)
- Modest response to β_2-agonist therapy.

Potentially life-threatening attack:
- Severe respiratory distress/retractions
- Unable to talk
- Exhaustion/confusion
- Cyanosis of lips or tongue (in room air)
- Silent chest/poor respiratory effort
- Marked tachypnoea and tachycardia
- Saturation <90% (if measured)
- Peak flow <33% predicted (if measured)
- No response to β_2-agonist therapy.

Treatment of chronic asthma

The various national guidelines describe four or five steps of escalating treatment (the number depending upon which side of the Atlantic they were composed) with the recommendation that the patient be started on the step most appropriate to the severity of the asthma. Most now recommend starting treatment on a step higher than would appear to be necessary and stepping down once control has been obtained. This implies an evaluation of severity, which has already been discussed, but it must be admitted that this can be difficult because many patients are already receiving some type of medication when referred for evaluation. In such a situation a reasonable 'guestimate' must be made of the overall asthma severity and the appropriate treatment step instituted. The differences between the adult and paediatric guidelines are fairly trivial and mainly involve the type of device for the inhalation of medications and the recommended doses.

Follow-up is essential to determine whether the current step is appropriate and whether treatment should be increased to the next step if inadequate or reduced if it appears to be set too high. Essential to this process of stepwise management is the evaluation of the adequacy of the control of asthma symptoms – the outcome guidelines.

Adequate control – no change in medication required:

- Minimal symptoms but not necessarily totally asymptomatic
- Minimal nocturnal asthma
- No limitation of everyday activities, no loss of work or schooling
- Occasional need for extra bronchodilator medication
- Able to exercise normally
- PEF >80% predicted or personal best (if being recorded at home)
- No side-effects from medications.

In the more severe asthmatics these ideals may not be achieved completely and the least possible symptoms and disturbance to everyday function will have to be accepted (steps 4 and 5 in the British guidelines – see below). As an extension of these outcome guidelines it is possible to suggest guidelines as to when treatment should be stepped up because of inadequate control or stepped down to test whether less treatment is required.

Inadequate control – increase medication:

- Daily symptoms or frequent nocturnal asthma
- Reduced everyday activities or some loss of work or schooling
- Daily need for extra bronchodilator medication

- PEF <80% predicted or personal best (if being recorded at home)
- Side-effects from medications may require change in medication.

Adequate control – try to reduce medication:

- No symptoms for at least 1–2 months
- No nocturnal asthma
- No limitation of everyday activities, no loss of work or schooling
- Able to exercise normally
- No need for extra bronchodilator medication
- PEF >80% predicted (if being recorded at home).

Guidelines for the pharmacological management of chronic asthma

The mainstay of treatment of asthma is the use of drugs to relieve airways obstruction and reduce the immunological inflammatory processes in the airways which cause bronchial hyperreactivity. The individual groups of drugs are considered more fully in other chapters. A simplified version of the five steps in the guidelines for the pharmacological management of childhood asthma are shown in **Figure 43** and amplified below. These apply to adults and children above about 2 years

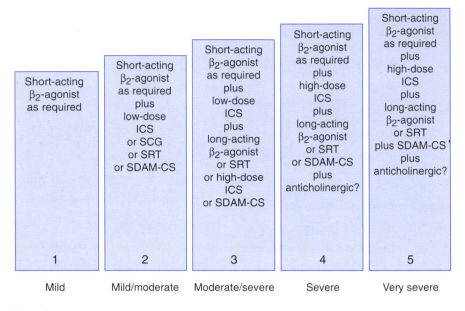

Figure 43
Steps in the management of chronic asthma in children and adults. For details and the management of the wheezy infant see text. ICS = inhaled corticosteroid; SCG = sodium cromoglycate or nedocromil sodium; SRT = slow-release theophylline; SDAM-CS = oral single-dose alternate-morning corticosteroid

of age because management of the wheezy infant is far less certain and indeed controversial and is considered later. Whatever step is decided upon it may be necessary to begin with a short 5–7 day course of oral corticosteroids at the start of treatment if the patient is significantly obstructed at the time.

A major factor in the management of asthma is the ability of the patient to take medications, especially inhaled medications, correctly. It is quite useless to prescribe a metered-dose inhaler without a spacer for the very young and the very elderly and quite unrealistic to expect parents to administer medications through a nebulizer to a screaming infant who is terrified by the noise of the compressor. The choice of inhalation device must be tailored to each patient and its efficient use ensured by education of the patient and family (and sometimes even the doctor). The most commonly used inhalation devices are discussed in **Chapter 5** and include the pressurized metered-dose inhaler (pMDI) alone or with some type of spacer holding chamber (pMDI-SP), the dry powder inhaler (DPI) and the jet nebulizer (NEB). The ultrasonic nebulizer is used much less often for the delivery of asthma medications.

Step 1: used for mild asthma: inhaled β_2-agonist as required:

- Use a short-acting β_2-agonist as required for symptom relief (1–2 puffs by pMDI or pMDI-SP usually)
- Oral preparations may be tried in young children but the inhaled route is more effective and much to be preferred for all patients
- If treatment is required more than once daily, move to step 2 after ensuring that patient indeed has a good inhaler technique.

Step 2: used for mild to moderate asthma: regular inhaled anti-inflammatory drugs:

- Use a short-acting inhaled β_2-agonist as required for symptom relief
- Add a regular anti-inflammatory agent as preventative (prophylactic) medication

- A low-dose inhaled corticosteroid is now the treatment of choice even by most paediatricians although some would use a cromone before moving to the corticosteroid
- Start with a higher dose (400–600 µg twice daily for BDP or budesonide, 200–300 µg for fluticasone) and reduce dose once control is achieved. Children may need lower doses.

Step 3: used for moderate to severe asthma: high-dose inhaled corticosteroids or low-dose corticosteroid together with a regular bronchodilator:

- Use a short-acting inhaled β_2-agonist as required for symptom relief
- Increased inhaled corticosteroids up to 2000 µg daily of beclomethasone or budesonide (and half this amount of fluticasone) for adults and about half this for children
- Alternatively, a regular twice daily inhaled long-acting β_2-agonist such as salmeterol or formoterol may be used on a continuous basis together with a lower dose of inhaled corticosteroid
- A relatively low dose of sustained release oral theophylline to give a blood level of about 10 µg/ml has also been shown to be an effective steroid sparing strategy and is an

alternative to the addition of a long-acting β_2-agonist.

Step 4: used for severe asthma: high-dose inhaled corticosteroids together with regular bronchodilator:

- Use a short-acting inhaled β_2-agonist as required for symptom relief increase inhaled corticosteroids up to 2000 µg daily of BDP or budesonide (and half this amount of fluticasone) for adults and about half this for children
- Add a regular twice daily inhaled long-acting β_2-agonist such as salmeterol or formoterol or alternatively try a relatively low dose of sustained release oral theophylline to give a blood level of about 10 µg/ml
- An inhaled anticholinergic such as ipratropium or oxitropium bromide may be combined with the β_2-agonist.

Step 5: used for severe asthma unresponsive to lesser treatment: regular alternate morning oral corticosteroids:

  Use a short-acting inhaled β_2-agonist as required for symptom relief
- Inhaled corticosteroids up to 2000 µg daily of beclomethasone or budesonide (and half this amount of fluticasone) for adults and about half this for children

- Regular twice daily inhaled long-acting β_2-agonist, such as salmeterol or formoterol, or alternatively try a relatively low dose of sustained-release oral theophylline to give a blood level of about 10 µg/ml
- Add a regular oral corticosteroid in the lowest possible dose that controls symptoms. It should be given as a single dose in the morning or preferably as a single dose every other morning, especially in children
- It may be possible to reduce the dose of the inhaled corticosteroid
- Other additional medications should be used as in step 4 as appropriate
- In patients requiring high doses of oral corticosteroids the addition of methotrexate, cyclosporin A or gold may be tried as a steroid-sparing device.

There are some patients, especially infants and very young children who require regular corticosteroids to control their asthma but in whom it is quite impossible to administer the drug effectively by inhalation. In such patients alternate morning oral corticosteroid therapy should be used until the patient can be trained to use an inhaler device correctly.

The position of the new anti-leukotriene drugs that are becoming available for treating asthma is not yet firmly established. It would appear that they are likely to be most useful in steps 2–4 of the guidelines either to replace low-dose inhaled cortico-steroids or to enable a lower dose of corticosteroid to be used.

Step-down: used once control has been achieved on a given step:

- Treatment should be reviewed every 1–2 months initially and at longer intervals as experience is gained with the individual patient
- Step-wise reduction of treatment may be possible if the patient has been virtually symptom free and requires little or no rescue additional bronchodilator medication for 1–2 months
- Patients with markedly seasonal variations in asthma severity may need to vary their treatment accord-ing to the season.

Treatment of acute severe asthma

Any patient with asthma of whatever grade can occasionally have an attack of acute, severe asthma which may or may not be so severe as to be life threatening as defined by the clinical features described earlier. Many patients coming to hospital with an acute severe attack of asthma have received little or no treatment and others have only been given extra doses of β_2-agonists in addition to their usual medication. Most studies of factors related to death from asthma have found inadequate treatment to be important and it has been estimated that about 40% of deaths could have been avoided by appropriate manage-ment. In most patients who die from asthma there is a background of chronic under-treatment for various reasons and inadequate management of the final episode is due about equally to delay on the part of the patient in seeking help and inadequate treatment by the physician. Even mild asthmatics can suffer an acute severe attack that kills them and in a survey from Australia it was found that about one-third of children who died from asthma were judged to have been mild asthmatics prior to the terminal illness.

The various guidelines which have been prepared for the management of asthma have also addressed the management of acute exacerbations. In some there are different recommenda-tions for management at home or in hospital which is useful. A simplified version of this two phase approach is

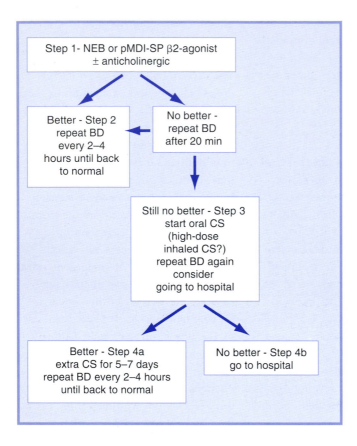

Figure 44
Ambulatory management of a non-life-threatening attack of asthma. For details see text. NEB = nebulizer; pMDI-SP = pressurized metered-dose inhaler with spacer; BD = bronchodilators (β_2-agonists ± anticholinergic); CS = corticosteroid

shown in **Figures 44 and 45** and amplified below.

The correct management of acute exacerbations of asthma depends upon:

For ambulatory patients:
• Correct interpretations of warning symptoms at home
• Correct treatment at home
• Recognition when hospital treatment is needed.

For patients coming to hospital:
• Correct evaluation in Accident and Emergency Department
• Correct treatment in Accident and Emergency Department

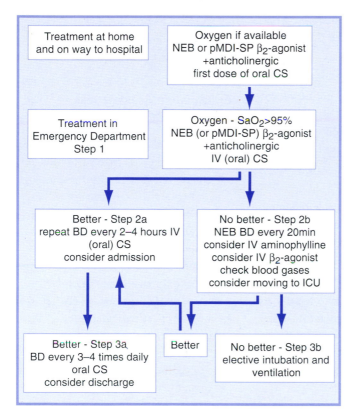

- Recognition when transfer to intensive care is needed
- Correct timing of discharge from hospital.

For all patients:
- Correct follow-up and modification of treatment.

Ambulatory treatment for non-life-threatening attack

Step 1

- Nebulized β_2-agonist bronchodilator if nebulizer available
- pMDI-SP β_2-agonist is good alternative

- Some add an anticholinergic bronchodilator to the β_2-agonist

Step 2
- Feeling better: repeat bronchodilator every 2–4 hours until back to usual state
- No better: repeat step 1 after 20 minutes and if still no better, move to:

Step 3
- Start oral corticosteroids (beginning of 5–7 day course) and repeat bronchodilator after 20 minutes

Step 4a
- If better, take extra bronchodilator as needed until back to usual state
- Some would recommend doubling dose of inhaled corticosteroid if being used as alternative to starting oral corticosteroid provided patient is not deteriorating

Step 4b
- If no better consider going straight to hospital or calling an ambulance

Treatment of potentially life-threatening attack

Treatment at home and on way to hospital
- Oxygen if available
- Nebulized β_2-agonist combined with anticholinergic if nebulizer available, or pMDI + spacer β_2-agonist and anticholinergic
- First dose of oral prednisolone

Evaluation in Accident And Emergency Department

- Quick history including medications already taken in past 24 hours
- Quick, relevant physical examination (cyanosis, retractions, air entry)
- Tachycardia and tachypnoea suggest severe asthma
- Bradycardia, hypotension suggest severe asthma
- Pulse oximetry – saturation <90% on room air suggests severe asthma
- Urgent chest radiograph if pneumothorax suspected but *don't delay treatment*
- Arterial blood gas analysis if asthma thought to be severe

Treatment in Accident and Emergency Department

Step 1
- Oxygen by face mask to keep saturation >95%
- Nebulized β_2-agonist combined with anticholinergic
- Oral prednisolone if patient relatively well and willing and able to swallow medications otherwise

intravenous methylprednisolone or hydrocortisone.

If the patient improves, progress to:

Step 2a

- Oxygen as needed
- Repeat bronchodilators every 2–4 hours
- Oral/intravenous corticosteroids once daily (6-hourly dosing is traditional but unnecessary)
- Monitor heart rate, respiratory rate and saturation.

Continuing improvement, progress to:

Step 3a

- Stop intravenous therapy
- Regular inhaled bronchodilators
- Oral corticosteroids once daily (twice daily dosing is traditional but unnecessary)
- Consider discharge and changes in regular medication.

If the patient does not improve after step 1, progress to:

Step 2b

- Add nebulized anticholinergic if not already being used
- Nebulized bronchodilators every 20 minutes
- Consider intravenous aminophylline (only maintenance dose if patient takes theophylline preparations at home). Measure theophylline level if aminophylline is being used

- Consider intravenous β_2-agonist
- Repeat blood gas measurement
- Measure electrolytes and glucose
- Beware of inappropriate ADH secretion – do not overload with fluids
- Consider moving the patient to intensive care unit (ICU) if:
  - Patient becoming tired with weak respiratory effort
  - Patient becoming comatosed
  - Arterial P_{O_2} <60 mmHg (<8 kPa) or saturation <90% on >60% inspired O_2
  - Arterial P_{CO_2} >45 mmHg (>6 kPa)

Step 3b

- Move to ICU before patient stops breathing
- Remember that elective intubation and ventilation is always better than an emergency procedure
- *Never give sedatives* unless the patient is intubated and ventilated
- Continue asthma medications while patient is being ventilated.

When the patient starts improving with or without a period of ventilation, continue with steps 2a and 3a.

Discharge from hospital after acute attack of asthma

When the patient has recovered sufficiently from the acute attack consideration must be given to the timing of discharge from hospital and what steps, if any, are needed for changes to management after discharge remembering that many patients were receiving inadequate treatment before admission. When the patient is symptom free or has returned more or less to the state that existed before the acute exacerbation, discharge can be considered. There should be good air entry without wheezing on examination and the PEF should be greater than 75% predicted or personal best if it can be measured. Oxygen saturation should be greater than 92% breathing room air. It is important to ensure that the patient and family have a full understanding of medications to be taken and the ability to use any prescribed inhaler device correctly. Medications that will be used after discharge should be started while in hospital and the patient should be observed to ensure that they are being taken correctly.

After admission to hospital for an acute attack of asthma, discharge medications should include a steadily reducing course of oral corticosteroids over about 1 week and regular inhaled bronchodilators until completely symptom free, then on an 'as needed' basis. If inhaled corticosteroids were being used before admission the dose should be increased

for 2–3 weeks. If regular prophylaxis was not being used before admission consideration should be given to starting this type of management if the overall asthma severity (see above) warrants it. However, an admission for an acute attack of asthma is not necessarily a reason for starting prophylaxis if the patient suffers from infrequent attacks. A written self-management 'action plan' describing the recommended treatment and the action to be taken when there is a change in well-being should be provided and it is sometimes helpful to supply an asthma diary with or without a peak-flow meter when there is doubt about the quality of the ambulatory control of the asthma.

Special problems in managing asthma

The wheezy infant

The wheezy infant presents one of the commonest and greatest diagnostic and management problems in paediatrics. In countries with well-defined seasons there is an epidemic of bronchiolitis in infants each winter that is usually due to infection with respiratory syncytial virus (RSV). The infection results in wheeze, cough and shortness of breath lasting for a few days and closely resembles an asthma attack clinically except that the airways obstruction is normally unresponsive to medications effective in children with asthma. There is no doubt that some children with asthma begin to wheeze in the first year or two of life and there is no doubt that many infants with acute viral bronchiolitis have recurrent attacks of wheezing after the initial illness. There is some evidence to suggest that the children who wheeze before the age of 3 years and stop wheezing are different from those who continue to wheeze and who are often atopic and with a family background of asthma. In a long-term controlled study of infants admitted to hospital at a mean age of 14 weeks with proven RSV bronchiolitis some 38% of the RSV group of infants had repeated episodes of mild wheezing during the first 4 years of life compared with 15% of the controls. However by the age of 10 years only 6.2% of the RSV group and 4.5% of the control group were wheezing. Clinically and physiologically, the bronchiolitic infant has marked airways obstruction with ventilation–perfusion mismatching and hypoxia. The chest X-ray may well be normal although non-specific infiltrates are not uncommon. Occasionally the infant may be very ill with marked hypoxia and may develop

respiratory failure, but this is quite unusual. The management of the infant with recurrent wheezing less than about 2 years of age is problematical. There is no doubt that a small proportion of such infants do indeed have asthma and respond well to the same medications as do older children. For such infants the guidelines described above are applicable with particular attention to the technique of administration of inhaled medications. However, many infants with recurrent wheezing are not true asthmatics and their disease is probably the result of temporary damage to the small airways following acute viral bronchiolitis. Given that at present the differential diagnosis of non-asthmatic post-bronchiolitic wheezing from infantile asthma is impossible on clinical and physiological grounds in most infants, the most logical approach in any chronically wheezy infant is to treat as if it were asthma using the guidelines described above. If there is a good clinical response, then the treatment should be continued as appropriate but if not, serious consideration should be given to withdrawal of any oral or inhaled corticosteroids that are being used. Most would inevitably continue to receive β_2-agonists but at least these are not likely to be harmful. It is also important to consider alternative diagnoses in the infant who does not respond.

Exercise-induced asthma (EIA)

While most asthmatics will develop a short attack of asthma as a result of physical exercise, this is commonest in fit adolescents and young adults who take part in vigorous sports. In these patients it may be the only troublesome manifestation of the disease. The problem can be avoided or dealt with by recommending appropriate types of exercise such as swimming or short duration intense exercise and by the appropriate use of medication of which the inhalation of a β_2-agonist just before exercise is the most effective therapy. EIA is due to the hyperventilation of exercise, which causes cooling and drying of the airway surface. This in turn may lead to the release of bronchoconstricting mediators from mast cells and the activation of sensory nerves, resulting in bronchoconstriction. EIA is most likely to occur when the exercise consists of 6–8 minutes of continuous hard exercise, breathing cool or dry air. If the patient is atopic, EIA is likely to be more troublesome during the allergy season. The conditions least likely to cause an attack of

EIA are intermittent exercise, for example many team games, swimming or other exercises breathing warm humid air. Asthmatics should be encouraged to take part in normal physical activities and use their β_2-agonist inhaler if necessary to enable them to compete on equal terms.

Nocturnal asthma

Nearly all asthmatics have worse asthma during the night than by day. This is often manifest in children by waking at night, coughing or wheezing, and in adults by waking early in the morning with chest tightness. This diurnal variation in asthma severity is very common and is a manifestation of airway hyperresponsiveness. Although the mechanism of nocturnal asthma is not completely understood, it may be related to circadian changes in circulating adrenaline and cortisol and vagal cholinergic tone. There is also evidence that airway inflammation and airway hyperresponsiveness increase at night. The best method of dealing with this problem is to give the patient effective anti-inflammatory medication throughout the 24 hours. If symptoms persist add either a long-acting inhaled β_2-agonist at night, or a slow-release theophylline preparation.

Aspirin- and NSAID-sensitive asthma

A very small proportion of asthmatics, almost always adults with relatively late-onset non-atopic asthma, are sensitive to aspirin and other NSAIDs. These patients commonly also have nasal polyps and perennial rhinitis. The ingestion of aspirin and other NSAIDs initially causes vasomotor rhinitis but later the patient responds to ingestion by developing an attack of asthma that may be very severe and even life-threatening. The mechanism involves increased production of bronchoconstricting leukotrienes by blockade of the cyclo-oxygenase pathway. It is important to enquire about the possible association of asthma attacks and NSAID ingestion, especially in adult-onset asthma, because these drugs are best avoided for life. Most such patients can tolerate paracetamol. Desensitization may be possible if NSAID therapy is essential, but this requires expert supervision. Anti-leukotrienes may be the treatment of choice for these patients.

Pregnancy

The effect of pregnancy on the woman with asthma is uncertain since in some the disease becomes easier to control,

in some it becomes more difficult, and in others there is no change. There are no means of predicting the response of the individual. None of the important drugs used to treat asthma, such as the β_2-agonists, sodium cromoglycate and inhaled corticosteroids, have been shown to have any adverse effect on the fetus or mother, while hypoxia is certainly bad for both. Every effort should be made to control asthma symptoms and maintain near normal lung function by the use of conventional medications, increasing the dose of inhaled corticosteroids if necessary. Oral corticosteroids can also be safely used when needed. On the whole, it is best to avoid adrenaline but this drug is rarely indicated. It is important to encourage pregnant women and mothers not to smoke, as there is good evidence that smoking increases the risk of developing asthma in infants. Smoking also causes fetal growth retardation, as well as adversely affecting the mother's asthma.

Gastro-oesophageal reflux (GOR)

GOR is not uncommon in infancy, even in the absence of any neurological disturbance, and the clinical picture of micro-aspiration may mimic asthma, with short episodes of reversible airways obstruction. This is distinct from massive aspiration, which causes pneumonia. There is considerable debate about the importance of GOR in older asthmatics, since some patients with particularly resistant asthma seem to benefit from anti-reflux medication or even surgery. Oral bronchodilators (β_2-agonists and theophylline) may increase acid reflux, and inhaled medication is preferred in patients with symptoms. A trial of effective anti-reflux therapy is indicated if there are symptoms (proton pump inhibitors, such as omeprazole and Iansoprozole, are more effective than H_2-antagonists, such as ranitidine).

Occupational asthma

Occupational asthma is a very special-ized field and full of pitfalls for those unaware of the important clinical and medico-legal ramifications. There is no doubt that some agents can cause asthma to develop in some individuals who have never before had the disease, and can make asthma worse in those that have. The latency period may be months or even years after first exposure, which makes diagnosis all the more difficult. Typically, the asthma will steadily deteriorate during the working week, only to get better when exposure ceases at the weekend or when on holiday. The symptomatic complaints should be checked by daily PEF measurement. When there appears to be a true link to a particular agent, a challenge test should be performed under controlled laboratory conditions that mimic the working conditions as closely as possible. The best treatment is to avoid the offending substance but the patient may also require regular anti-asthma medication. It is not uncommon for the asthma to persist even after leaving the workplace.

Brittle 'catastrophic' asthma

One of the less common types of asthma is that in which the patient suffers from sudden, devastatingly severe attacks, which may occur against a background of apparently normal health. These patients are at risk from dying suddenly and should be treated with the utmost care. They should always carry emergency supplies of medications plus the necessary equip-ment to effectively administer a high dose of β_2-agonist (MDI with or without spacer), and a supply of oral corticos-teroids that should be swallowed at the first sign of deterioration. Some patients may need to carry self-injectable adrena-line if the attacks develop so rapidly or are so severe that inhaled medication is of no value. The patient should always carry written instructions about emergency treatment and, if possible, a warning bracelet in case he or she is unable to administer medications. Some patients with frequent marked variations in PEF may be helped by subcutaneous β_2-agonist infusions (via insulin pump). Many would place this type of patient on continuous anti-inflammatory treatment even though their attacks are often infrequent.

Corticosteroid-resistant asthma

Some asthmatics, mostly adults but occasionally children or adolescents, appear to be resistant to all forms of conventional medication, including corticosteroid therapy (**Figure 46**). In such patients, it is important to be sure that they do indeed have asthma and not some other condition, such as cystic fibrosis, GOR, bronchiolitis obliterans or emphysema, and it is equally important to be sure that they are taking their prescribed medications correctly and regularly. In the majority of such patients there will be a simple technical reason to explain the poor response, such as poor inhaler technique, poor compliance with treatment, or emotional disturbance. All

apparently resistant patients should be given a trial of oral corticosteroids (prednisolone 40–60 mg daily for 2 weeks in adults) which also provides the opportunity to check compliance by measurement of diurnal cortisol levels and plasma prednisolone levels (when available). Sometimes these patients may respond to parenteral depot corticosteroid preparations, such as triamcinolone acetonide and this may also serve as a check on patient compliance with treatment.

True corticosteroid resistance is very rare and appears to be due to an abnormality in the interaction between the glucocorticoid receptor and DNA. A more common occurrence is relative resistance, when patients require high doses of oral corticosteroid to control their asthma. This may be helped by steroid-sparing therapies such as methotrexate, oral gold, or cyclosporin A. Long-acting inhaled β_2-agonists and theophylline may be helpful in these patients; anti-leukotrienes may also be beneficial.

Patient education and doctor–patient relationships: living with asthma

The successful management of asthma depends to a very large degree on

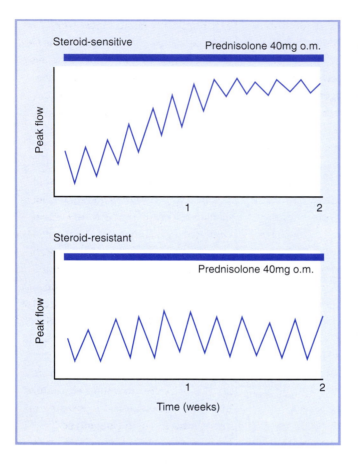

Figure 46
*Corticosteroid-resistant
asthma is defined as a
lack of clinical response to
prednisolone 30–40 mg
daily over 2 weeks,
providing that the treatment
is adhered to*

providing the patient with a good understanding of the nature of asthma and its treatment. The physician must take time to explain this to the patient in terms that he or she (or the parents of a small child) can understand, and the message must be reinforced at subsequent visits. It needs to be explained that there is no cure for asthma but there is excellent treatment that can allow virtually all asthmatics to lead normal lives. There may be long-term or even permanent remissions of the disease, especially in children and there are data to show that about two-thirds of children apparently 'grow out' of their asthma completely. The long-term prognosis is less certain in adults with asthma but at all ages there is accumulating evidence that effective anti-inflammatory treatment improves the prognosis and helps avoid irreparable damage to the airways. Asthma is rarely fatal but in those cases where it is, there has almost always been inadequate treatment or failure to comply with medical advice. In particular it is important to emphasize that far more patients die because they do not get corticosteroid therapy than the reverse. In conventional doses, corticosteroids are not harmful to either children or adults and they form the mainstay of the treatment of serious chronic asthma at all ages.

Compliance

Compliance (or adherence) with treatment is essential and the major causes of inadequate control of asthma and consequent suffering are the 3 Fs:

- Failure to take prescribed medications regularly
- Failure to take the prescribed dose
- Failure to use inhalers properly.

The physician should make every attempt to verify compliance with treatment at each visit and should always check on inhaler technique and the functioning of spacer devices. The simpler the regimen, the more likely is patient compliance and successful control of asthma.

Teachers and other care-givers should be able to deal with asthmatic children in their care since at least 10–15% of the class are likely to have asthma. This means that they should know which children in their class have asthma, something about the nature of the disease and its treatment. In particular they should appreciate that exercise can be difficult for the asthmatic child who may need to take a β_2-agonist before exercise. They should also be able to recognize deteriorating asthma in a pupil and inform the parents and know how to administer inhaled medications for an acute attack. It is self-evident that teachers and other role models should not smoke and should strongly discourage smoking by children, especially asthmatics.

Ancillary devices to aid management

Diaries and PEF meters. Given the fact that the management of asthma is ambulatory for most patients almost all of the time, the physician often needs objective information on the condition of the patient while engaged in normal activities. The patient also needs to know what to do about his or her treatment without consulting the physician at every turn. A number of ancillary devices have been developed for these purposes. The simplest and possibly the most useful device is a daily record of symptoms and drug consumption. The patient is asked to fill in a card each day to record the intensity of nocturnal and daytime symptoms and the number of doses of all medications consumed. These diaries are particularly useful when evaluating a new patient, or when changing treatment regimens. They also provide a useful check on patient compliance. The ambulatory monitoring of lung function can be undertaken by using a simple PEF meter twice daily at home and this was originally introduced as an addendum to the diary score. In recent years, great emphasis has been placed on the continuous use of PEF meters at home by all chronic asthmatics, with treatment guidelines being based on some defined value of PEF or its diurnal variation. In truth, all but the most obsessive patients find this irksome and most soon abandon regular recording. There

is no doubt that all patients whose asthma is difficult to control should record their PEF twice daily but the need for this in well-controlled patients is less certain.

Actions plans. A further extension of the diary and PEF recording is to provide the patient with a written 'Action plan' detailing the recommended treatment. There are a wide variety of these, stretching from the simple and practical to those requiring a college degree and a computer for their use! As with all asthma management – the simpler the better. If the action plan occupies more than one typed sheet it will probably not be understood by most patients and its recommendations will not be obeyed. The action plan should contain the name and telephone number of all treating physicians/hospitals, how the patient should feel when well controlled based on symptoms and/or PEF recording, when to take extra medications and how much to take and how to step down treatment when condition improves.

Further reading

Asthma: a follow up statement from an international paediatric asthma consensus group. *Arch Dis Child* (1992); **67:** 240–8.

British Thoracic Society and others (1997) The British guidelines on asthma management 1995 review and position statement. *Thorax* **52**(Suppl 1): S1–21.

Expert Panel Report 2 (1997) Guidelines for the diagnosis and management of asthma. Publication 97-4051. National Institutes of Health, Washington, DC.

Global Initiative for Asthma (1995) Global strategy for asthma management and prevention. NHLBI/WHO Workshop Report, Publication 95–3659.

New treatments for asthma

7

Improved understanding of asthma has led to the development of several new treatments for asthma. Currently available therapy for asthma is highly effective and, if use appropriately, there are usually no problems with adverse effects. However, some patients (~5–10% of asthmatic patients) remain poorly controlled, despite what appears to be optimal therapy. There are some concerns about the safety of asthma therapy, particularly in the treatment of childhood asthma, as this treatment has to be given over a very long period. Compliance with inhaled therapy, particularly controller therapy, is poor and might be improved with oral therapy (once-daily calender pack). Yet oral therapy presents a problem of side-effects since the drug exerts effects throughout the body, whereas asthma is localized to the airways. This will necessitate the development of drugs that are *specific* for asthma and do not have effects on other systems or on normal physiological mechanisms (unlike β-agonists and glucocorticoids). None of the currently available therapy is curative or has so far been shown to alter the natural history of the disease. Perhaps it is difficult to seek a cure for asthma until more is known about the molecular causes.

Despite considerable efforts by the pharmaceutical industry it has been very difficult to develop new classes of therapeutic agent. Asthma is the most rapidly growing therapeutic market in the world, reflecting the world-wide increase in prevalence of asthma and the increasing recognition that chronic treatment is needed for many patients. It is clearly important to understand more about the underlying mechanisms of asthma and also about how the currently used drugs work before ratio-nal improvements in therapy can be expected. There are several opportuni-ties for new drug development in asthma, but whether these will revolu-tionize asthma treatment is unknown.

There are three major approaches to the development of new anti-asthma treatments:
- Improvement in existing classes of effective drug, e.g. long-acting β_2-agonists (salmeterol and formoterol), or long-acting anticholinergics (tiotropium bromide)
- Development of novel compounds, based on rational developments and improved understanding of asthma, e.g. anti-leukotrienes or IL-5 inhibitors
- Development of novel compounds based on serendipity, e.g. frusemide.

New bronchodilators

Bronchodilators are presumed to act by reversing contraction of airway smooth muscle, although some may have additional effects on mucosal oedema or inflammatory cells. The biochemical basis of airway smooth muscle relaxation has been studies extensively, yet no new types of bronchodilator have had any clinical impact. The molecular basis of bronchodilatation involves an increase in intracellular cAMP and a reduction in cytosolic calcium ion concentration ($[Ca^{2+}]$) (**Figure 47**). Recent studies suggest that the rise in cAMP is linked to the opening of certain potassium (K^+) channels in airway smooth muscle. Also β-agonists may open K^+ channels via a direct G-protein coupling to the channel, and this may occur at low concentra-tions of β-agonist that do not involve any increase in cAMP concentration. The molecular mechanisms underlying bronchodilatation may be exploited in the development of new bronchodila-tors, several of which are under develop-ment (**Table 7**).

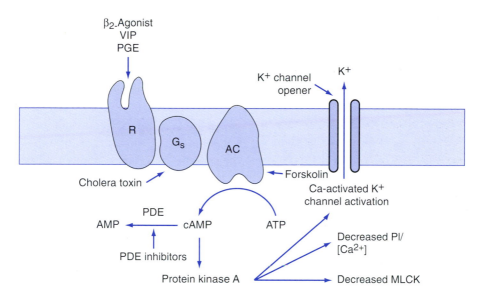

Figure 47
New bronchodilators based on the mechanism of action of β₂-agonists

Table 7
New bronchodilators.

- Long-acting inhaled β₂-agonists (e.g. salmeterol, formoterol)
- Novel xanthine derivatives
- Selective muscarinic antagonists (M_1/M_3 antagonists under development, e.g. tiotropium)
- Potassium channel activators (e.g. levcromakalim)
- Selective phosphodiesterase inhibitors
- Nitrovasodilators
- VIP and analogues
- Atrial natriuretic peptide and analogues (urodilatin)

β₂-Agonists

Long-acting inhaled β₂-agonists (salmeterol and formoterol) have been an important clinical development, and it is theoretically possible to develop drugs with an even longer duration of action that are suitable for once daily dosing. It is unlikely that development of drugs more selective for β-receptors would have any advantage.

Other drugs that increase cyclic AMP

Understanding the molecular mechanism of β-agonists has prompted a search for other drugs that increase intracellular cAMP concentrations in airway smooth muscle cells. These drugs include:

- *Vasoactive intestinal peptide* (VIP): a potent bronchodilator of human airways in vitro, but is ineffective in asthmatic patients due to breakdown by enzymes. Even stable analogues, such as Ro-25-1553 are unlikely to be useful as they are potent vasodilators and would cause side-effects, such as headaches, flushing and postural hypotension
- *Prostaglandin E*: is also a bronchodilator in vitro, but is unsuitable as a treatment as it induces coughing

- *Selective phosphodiesterase (PDE) inhibitors* that inhibit the breakdown of cAMP by PDEs, of which many different types have now been characterized. Some PDEs are more important in smooth muscle relaxation, with the predominance of PDE_3 in human airway smooth muscle. However, PDE_3 inhibitors have been associated with cardio-vascular abnormalities, particularly arrhythmias, and it is unlikely that they would have a safety profile that would allow their clinical development.

Drugs that increase cyclic GMP

Cyclic GMP, like cAMP also relaxes human airway smooth muscle, but drugs that increase cGMP also relax vascular smooth muscle so are prone to vasodilator side-effects.

Atrial natriuretic peptide (ANP) is a bronchodilator, but as it is a peptide it is expensive and is not absorbed after oral administration. Urodilatin is an extended form of ANP that is less susceptible to degradation by enzymes and is being developed as a bronchodilator particularly for exacerbations of asthma.

New anticholinergics

There has been a search for anticholinergics that are more selective for certain subtypes of muscarinic receptors – specifically the M_3-receptor that mediates the bronchoconstrictor effects of cholinergic nerves. Although some selective drugs have been identified they do not have a degree of selectivity that gives them any clinical advantage. However, a new important development is the discovery of a long-acting inhaled anticholinergic, tiotropium bromide, which only needs to be given once a day. Its main indication will be in the treatment of COPD.

K⁺ channel openers

When K^+ channels are opened, relaxation of smooth muscle results and drugs that selectively activate K^+ channels in smooth muscle have now been developed. One such drug is levcromakalim, which is a potent relaxant of human airways in vitro. When given to asthmatic patients, however, levcromakalim has no bronchodilator action or protective effect against bronchoconstrictor challenge at maximally tolerated oral doses. Levcromakalim is a potent vasodilator and gives side-effects such as headaches, flushing and postural hypotension. By inhalation these vasodilator effects are not avoided as the drug is absorbed from the lung.

Mediator antagonists

Many different inflammatory mediators have now been implicated in asthma, and several specific receptor antagonists and synthesis inhibitors have been developed that will prove invaluable in working out the contribution of each mediator (**Table 8**). As many mediators probably contribute to the pathological features of asthma, it seems unlikely that a single antagonist will have a major clinical effect, compared with non-specific agents such as β-agonists and glucocorticoids. However, until such drugs have been evaluated in careful clinical studies, it is not possible to predict their value. Most of the mediator antagonists when tested in asthmatic patients have been very disappointing, despite promising results in animal models of experimental asthma. The drugs that have now been shown to be clinically useful so far include thromboxane antagonists and synthase inhibitors, platelet-activating factor antagonists, bradykinin antagonists, antihistamines and

Table 8
Inflammatory mediator inhibitors.

Mediator	Inhibitor
Histamine	Terfenadine, loratadine, cetirizine
Leukotriene D_4	Zafirlukast, montelukast, zileuton, Bay-x1005, ZD 2138
Leukotriene B_4	LY 293111
PAF	Apafant, modipafant, bepafant
Thromboxane	Ozagrel
Bradykinin	Icatibant, WIN 64338
Adenosine	Theophylline
Reactive oxygen species	N-acetyl-cysteine, ascorbic acid, nitrones
Nitric oxide	Aminoguanidine, 1400W
Endothelin	Bosentan, SB 209670
IL-1β	Recombinant IL-1 receptor antagonist
TNF-α	TNF-antibody, TNF soluble receptors
IL-4	IL-4 antibody
IL-5	IL-5 antibody
Mast cell tryptase	APC366
Eosinophil basic proteins	Heparin

tachykinin antagonists. The only class of drugs that has been shown to have a useful clincial effect are anti-leukotrienes (leukotrienes receptor antagonists and 5'-lipoxygenase inhibitors), as discussed in **Chapter 4**. Some antagonists which have not yet been tested properly in asthma include inhibitors of inducible nitric oxide synthase (which generates large amounts of nitric oxide in asthma), effective antioxidants and cytokine inhibitors.

Cytokines and cytokine inhibitors

A complex cytokine network is responsible for maintaining the chronic inflammation in asthma, as discussed in **Chapter 1**. Amongst the many cytokines involved in asthma, some may be more important in determining the nature of the inflammatory response or in amplifying the inflammatory state. There are several possible approaches to inhibiting specific cytokines (**Figure 48**). These range from drugs that inhibit

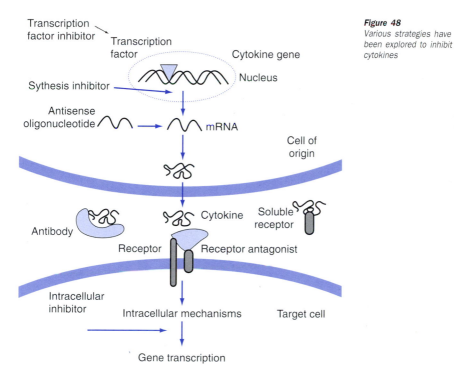

Figure 48
Various strategies have been explored to inhibit cytokines

cytokine synthesis (e.g. corticosteroids, cyclosporin A), blocking antibodies to cytokines or their receptors, soluble receptors to mop up secreted cytokines, receptor antagonists or drugs that block the signal transduction pathways activated by cytokines. Other cytokines appear to have an anti-inflammatory effect and may therefore be regarded as potentially therapeutic.

IL-5 plays a key role in orchestrating the eosinophilic inflammation of asthma. Blocking antibodies to IL-5 have been shown to inhibit eosinophilic inflammation and airway hyperresponsiveness in animal models of asthma, including primates and this blocking effect may last for up to 3 months after a single injection. This makes treatment of chronic asthma with such a therapy a feasible proposition. Humanized antibodies have now been developed and are in clinical trial in asthma. There is also a search for IL-5 receptor antagonists.

IL-4 is critical for the synthesis of IgE by B-lymphocytes and is also involved in eosinophil recruitment to the airways. Inhibition of IL-4 may therefore be effective in inhibiting allergic diseases, and anti-IL-4 receptors are now in clinical development as a strategy to inhibit IL-4.

TNF-α is expressed in asthmatic airways and may play a key role in amplifying asthmatic inflammation, through the activation of NF-κB and other transcription factors. In rheumatoid arthritis blocking antibodies to TNF-α have produced remarkable clinical benefits, even in patients who were relatively unresponsive to corticosteroids. Such antibodies or soluble TNF-receptors are a logical approach to asthma therapy, particularly in patients with severe disease. One problem encountered in this therapy is the development of antibodies that may limit the therapeutic effects after repeated administration, however.

Certain chemokines, such as RANTES and eotaxin, may play a critical role in the recruitment of eosinophils into the airways of asthmatic patients (see **Chapter 1**). Fortunately all of these chemokines act on a common receptor, the CCR3 receptor, that is expressed predominantly on eosinophils. It is possible that non-peptide inhibitors will be discovered by random screening of chemical libraries.

Some cytokines appear to have anti-inflammatory effects in asthmatic inflammation and may therefore be considered potentially therapeutic. While it may not be feasible to administer these proteins as long-term therapy, it may be possible to develop drugs that activate the same receptors or specific signal transduction pathways activated by these receptors. Interferon-γ (IFN-γ) inhibits Th$_2$ cells and should therefore theoretically reduce asthmatic inflammation. Administration of IFN-γ by nebulization to asthmatic patients has not been found to be very effective, however, possibly due to the difficulty in obtaining a high enough concentration locally in the airways. IL-12 is the endogenous regulator of Th$_1$ cells and determines the balance between Th$_1$ and Th$_2$ cells. IL-12 administration to animals inhibits allergen-induced inflammation and sensitization to allergens and is therefore a potential treatment for asthma that may reset a fundamental immunological switch. IL-10 inhibits the synthesis of many inflammatory cytokines that are overexpressed in asthma. Its effects are partly mediated via inhibition of NF-κB and is a potential therapy.

Anti-inflammatory drugs

There has been an intensive search for anti-inflammatory treatments that are as effective as glucocorticoids but with fewer side-effects. Several anti-inflammatory drugs for asthma are now in clinical development (**Table 9**).

New corticosteroids

Corticosteroids are the most efficacious treatment currently available for the long-term management of asthma and topical steroids, such as BDP, budesonide and fluticasone propionate are now widely used in asthma therapy. In order to reduce systemic effects further it may be necessary to increase the metabolism of any absorbed corticosteroid in the circulation, such as by erythrocyte-derived enzymes. It is important to prevent rapid metabolism in lung tissue as this appears to reduce anti-inflammatory action, as illustrated by the poor efficacy of the 'soft' corticosteroids butixocort and tipredane. Because corticosteroids are so effective in the control of asthma, an important goal of research is to identify the particular cellular and molecular mechanisms that are of critical importance in controlling asthmatic inflammation. It is now recognized that anti-inflammatory

Table 9
New anti-inflammatory drugs for asthma.

- New glucocorticoids (mometasone, cyclesonide, RP 106541)
- Immunomodulators (inhaled oxeclosporin, tacrolimus, rapamycin, mycophenolate mofetil)
- PDE_4 inhibitors (CDP 840, RP 73401, SB 207499)
- Adhesion molecule blockers (VLA-4 antibody)
- Cytokine inhibitors (anti-IL-4, anti-IL-5, anti-TNF antibodies)
- Anti-inflammatory cytokines (IL-1ra, IFN-γ, IL-10, IL-12)
- Anti-IgE antibody
- Peptides for immunotherapy

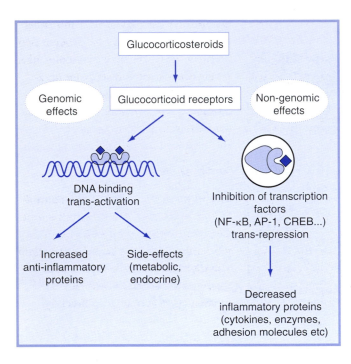

Figure 49
It may be possible to reduce the systemic side-effects of corticosteroids by designing drugs that lead to inhibition of transcription factors (anti-inflammatory effect) but do not lead to DNA binding (side-effects from the metabolic and endocrine actions of corticosteroids)

effects of glucocorticoids are likely to be via direct inhibition of transcription factors, such as activator protein-1 (AP-1) and NF-κB, that are activated by inflammatory signals, as discussed in **Chapter 3**. New corticosteroids that have a more potent effect on these mechanisms than on the classical mechanism of corticosteroid action which is likely to underlie systemic side-effects have now been discovered (**Figure 49**).

PDE$_4$ inhibitors

PDE$_4$ is the predominant PDE in the inflammatory cells involved in asthma, including mast cells, eosinophils, T-lymphocytes, macrophages, sensory nerves and epithelial cells (**Table 10**). This has suggested that PDE$_4$ inhibitors would be useful in asthma therapy as an anti-inflammatory treatment (**Figure 50**). In animal models of asthma, several PDE$_4$ inhibitors have been

Table 10
Distribution of phosphodiesterases in the airways.

Cell type	Predominant PDE isoenzymes
Smooth Muscle	
Airway smooth muscle	3, 4, 5
Vascular smooth muscle	3, 5
Inflammatory Cells	
Mast cell	4
Macrophage	4, 3
Monocyte	4
Eosinophil	4
Neutrophil	4
Platelet	3, 5
T-lymphocyte	4
Endothelial cell	3, 4
Sensory nerves	4
Airway epithelial cells	4

shown to reduce eosinophil inflammation and to reduce airway hyperresponsiveness. However, clinical studies have so far proved to be disappointing as nausea and vomiting, due to PDE_4 inhibition, are common and limit the dose of drug that can be given.

Anti-allergic drugs

Cromones may be effective in controlling mild asthma in some patients, but they are weak and the molecular mechanism of action remains uncertain. The diuretic frusemide (furosemide) shares many of the actions of cromones, in inhibiting indirect

- **Selective inhibitors:**
  - RP 73401, Org 20241, CDP840

- **Mixed inhibitors:**
  - Zardaverine, benafentrine, Org 30029

- **Anti-inflammatory**
  - Mast cells: decreased mediator release
  - Macrophages: decreased mediator/cytokine release
  - Eosinophils: decreased mediator release
  - T-lymphocytes: decreased cytokine release
  - Epithelial cells: decreased cytokine release
  - In vivo: decreased allergen-induced eosinophilic inflammation

- **Bronchodilator**
  Reverse induced tone

Figure 50
Phosphodiesterase 4 inhibitors may have anti-inflammatory and bronchodilator effects in asthma

bronchoconstrictor challenges (allergen, exercise, cold air) but not direct bronchoconstriction (histamine, methacholine) when given by inhalation. The mechanism of action of frusemide is not shared by other diuretics in the same class, suggesting that some mechanism other than their diuretic action must be involved. This is most likely to involve inhibition of the chloride channel that is also inhibited by cromones. Frusemide itself does not appear to be very effective when given regularly by metered-dose inhaler in asthma, but it is possible that more potent and long-lasting chloride-channel blockers might be developed in the future.

Immunomodulators

T-lymphocytes may play a critical role in initiating and maintaining the inflammatory process in asthma via the release of cytokines that result in eosinophilic inflammation, suggesting that T-cell inhibitors (immunomodulators) may be useful in controlling asthmatic inflammation. Glucocorticoids suppress inflammation in asthma partly through an inhibitory action on T-cell cytokine production. PDE_4 inhibitors also have an inhibitory action on T-cell function, and inhibit the secretion of

IL-5 from allergen-driven T-cells. Cyclosporin A may have a small corticosteroid-sparing effect in corticosteroid-dependent asthmatic patients, but its efficacy is limited, and side-effects, particularly nephrotoxicity, limit its widespread use. The problem of side-effects might be overcome by using the inhaled route of delivery. Novel immunomodulators, such as *mycophenolate mofetil*, may be less toxic and therefore of greater potential value in asthma therapy.

One problem with non-specific immunomodulators, such as cyclosporin A, is that they inhibit both Th_1 and Th_2 cells, and therefore do not rest the imbalance between these types of T-cell. They also inhibit suppressor T-cells that may modulate the inflammatory response. What is required is selective inhibition of Th_2 cells and there is now a search for such drugs.

Cell-adhesion blockers

The infiltration of inflammatory cells into tissues is dependent on specific adhesion molecules on both leukocytes and on endothelial cells. Antibodies which inhibit these adhesion molecules therefore may prevent inflammatory cell infiltration. Thus a monoclonal antibody to ICAM-1 on endothelial cells prevents the eosinophil infiltration into airways and the increase in bronchial reactivity after allergen exposure in sensitized primates. The interaction between VLA-4 and VCAM-1 is important for eosinophil inflammation and humanized antibodies to VLA-4 have now been developed. While blocking adhesion molecules is an attractive new approach to the treatment of inflammatory disease, there may be potential dangers in inhibiting immune responses leading to increased numbers of infections and increased risks of neoplasia.

IgE inhibition

Since release of mediators in asthma may be IgE-dependent, an alternative approach is to block the activation of IgE using blocking antibodies that do not result in cell activation. Anti-IgE antibodies have been developed that inhibit allergen-induced mast cell degranulation. Clinical studies in asthma show that it has some inhibitory effect in allergen-induced responses. While infusions of antibody may not be feasible for the long-term treatment of mild asthma, this could be a realistic therapy for patients with more severe forms of asthma. It may be possible to develop smaller

molecules in the future which inhibit IgE.

Eosinophil inhibitors

Several new drugs for asthma are aimed selective blockade of eosinophils. Indeed, there is unlikely to be any major side-effects for such a therapeutic approach. Eosinophil infiltration into the airways and their activation may be blocked in several ways (**Figure 51**). Eosinophil recruitment from the circulation may be blocked by antibodies to the adhesion molecules VCAM-1 (expressed on endothelial cells) and VLA-4 (expressed on eosinophils). Humanized VLA antibodies are not in clinical trial in asthma and small molecules that may be suitable for oral absorption are also in development. IL-5 plays an important role in eosinophil recruitment and selective blockade of IL-5 may therefore be a valuable approach. Humanized IL-5 antibodies are now in clinical trial in asthma, but other approaches to blocking IL-5 such as transcription blockade and inhibitors of IL-5 receptors are now under investigation. Chemokines play a critical role in selectively attracting eosinophils into the airways. As discussed above, although several chemokines (RANTES,

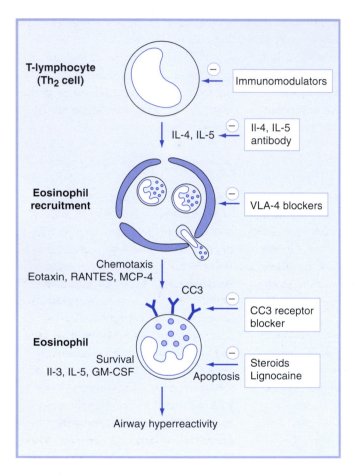

Figure 51
*Strategies for inhibiting
eosinophil inflammation*

MCP-4, eotaxin) are selective for eosinophils they all work through a common receptor on the eosinophil, CCR-3. Since this is a typical G-protein-coupled receptor with seven transmembrane-spanning domains, it may be possible to screen for CCR3 inhibitors. Once recruited into the airways, eosinophils would normally undergo programmed cell death (apoptosis), but survive due to the effects of various growth factors, such as IL-3, IL-5 and

GM-CSF. Corticosteroids induce eosinophil cell death, but other drugs may also have such an effect and the complex biochemical pathways involved in apoptosis may provide opportunities for selective eosinophil deletion.

Immunotherapy

Although immunotherapy as currently practised has been disappointing in the therapy of asthma, it is likely that more effective vaccines will be developed in the future. As the complex mechanisms of antigen presentation and the interaction between antigen-presenting cells and T-lymphocyte receptors are elucidated this may lead to the development of peptides that will block allergen-induced immune reactions. Such peptides are now in clinicial trials in allergic diseases.

Vaccination

The vast majority of asthma is allergic and allergy appears to be related to an imbalance between Th_1 and Th_2 cells. The development of allergic disease may be determined early in life by factors that affect this balance. There is a strong inverse association between a positive tuberculin test (indicating a Th_1-mediated response) and atopy. This suggests that it might be possible to immunize children against the risk of developing allergic diseases by stimulating local Th_1-mediated immunity in the respiratory tract before sensitization occurs.

Future trends in therapy

Many different therapeutic approaches to the treatment of asthma may be possible, yet there have been few new drugs that have reached the clinic. β-Agonists are by far the most effective bronchodilator drugs and lead to rapid symptomatic relief. Now that inhaled β_2-agonists with a long duration of action have been developed it is difficult to imagine that more effective bronchodilators could be discovered. Similarly, inhaled corticosteroids are extremely effective as chronic treatment in asthma and suppress the underlying inflammatory process. There is increasing evidence that earlier use of inhaled glucocorticoids may not only control asthma effectively, but may also prevent irreversible changes in airway function. For most patients a short-acting β_2-agonist on demand and regular inhaled corticosteroids are sufficient to give excellent control of asthma. For some patients a fixed combination β$_2$-agonist and cortico-steroid inhaler may be a useful development, since they will improve the compliance of inhaled corticosteroids (which is poor because of the lack of immediate bronchodilator effect).

The *ideal* drug for asthma would probably be a tablet that can be administered once daily to improve compliance. It should have no side-effects and this means that it should be specific for the abnormality of asthma (or allergy).

Future developments in asthma therapy should be directed towards the inflammatory mechanisms and perhaps more specific therapy may one day be developed. The possibility of developing a 'cure' for asthma seems remote, but when more is known about the genetic abnormalities of asthma it may be possible to search for such a therapy. Advances in molecular biology may aid the development of drugs that can specifically switch off relevant genes, but more must be discovered about the basic mechanisms of asthma before such advances are possible.

Further reading

Barnes PJ (1996) New drugs for asthma. *Clin Exp Allergy* **26:** 738–45.

Appendix: Doses of anti-asthma therapies

Bronchodilators

Salbutamol

Short-acting inhaled β_2-agonist for symptom relief
Syrup for small children: 0.15 mg/kg/dose (max
3 mg) up to 4 times daily
Nebulizer solution (5 mg/ml): 0.5 ml diluted to
2–3 ml up to 4 times daily
MDI (100 μg/puff) with or without spacer: 1–2 puffs
as needed up to 4 times daily
DPI (Diskhaler/Diskus): 200 or 400 μg, 1–2 inhala-
tions as needed up to 4 times daily
DPI (Easyhaler) 100 or 200 μg/dose
1–2 inhalations as needed up to 1600 μg daily
Slow-release tablet: 8 mg (4 mg in children) twice daily

Terbutaline

Short-acting inhaled β_2-agonist for symptom relief
Syrup for small children: 0.15 mg/kg/dose (max
3 mg) up to 4 times daily
Nebulizer solution (10 mg/ml): 0.5 ml diluted to
2–3 ml up to 4 times daily

	MDI (250 µg/puff) with or without spacer: 1–2 puffs as needed up to 4 times daily DPI (Turbohaler): (500 µg/dose; 200 µg/dose available on some markets); 1 inhalation up to 4 times daily
Fenoterol	Short-acting inhaled β_2-agonist for symptom relief MDI (100 µg/puff): 1–2 puffs as needed up to 4 times daily MDI (200 µg/puff): only indicated occasionally
Salmeterol	Long-acting inhaled β_2-agonist for regular use MDI (25 µg/puff): 1–2 puffs twice daily DPI (Diskhaler/Diskus): (50 µg/puff): 1–2 puffs twice daily
Formoterol (eformoterol fumarate)	Long-acting inhaled β_2-agonist for regular use DPI (12 µg/capsule): 1–2 capsules twice daily DPI (Turbohaler): 6–12 µg twice daily
Bambuterol	Long-acting oral β_2-agonist 10–20 mg at bedtime
Other β_2-agonists	Pirbuterol, reproterol, orciprenaline, rimiterol These are used less often

Note: It is not recommended to prescribe regular daily short-acting β_2-agonist medication on a long-term basis and these drugs should be used primarily as rescue medication. Salmeterol should only be used in combination with inhaled steroids.

Ipratropium bromide	Anticholinergic bronchodilator, less effective than β_2-agonists in routine asthma treatment Nebulizer solution (250 µg/ml): 0.25-1.00 ml 3-4 times daily MDI (20/40 µg/puff): 1-2 puffs 3-4 times daily DPI (40 µg/capsule): 1-2 capsules 3-4 times daily
Oxitropium bromide	MDI (100 µg/puff): 2 puffs 3 times daily
Combination bronchodilator inhalers	Combivent: MDI: ipratropium bromide (20 µg) and salbutamol (100 µg): 2 puffs 4 times daily Nebulizer: ipratropium bromide (500 µg) and salbutamol (2.5 mg) in 2.5 ml 3-4 times daily Duovent: MDI: ipratropium bromide (20 µg) and fenoterol (100 µg): 1-2 puffs 3-4 times daily Nebulizer: ipratropium bromide (500 µg) and salbutamol (1.25 mg) in 4 ml 3-4 times daily

Inhaled corticosteroids

Low-dose (BDP): total daily dose <800 µg in adults, 400 µg in children
High-dose (BDP): 800–2000 µg in adults, 400–1000 µg in children

- Dose delivered to lungs depends on delivery device
- Daily dose determined by asthma severity; use lowest dose needed to maintain control
- Twice daily administration recommended

Beclomethasone dipropionate

MDI (50, 100, 200 and 250 µg/puff)
DPI (Diskhaler) 100, 200 or 400 µg/dose
DPI (100, 200 and 400 µg/dose)
DPI (Easyhaler) 200 µg/dose

Budesonide

MDI (50 and 200 µg/puff)
DPI (Turbohaler) 100, 200 and 400 µg/inhalation
Nebulizer (250 µg/ml; 500 µg/ml)
1–2 mg twice daily

Fluticasone propionate

MDI (25, 50, 125 and 250 µg puff)
DPI (50, 100, 250 and 500 µg/dose)
Approximately twice as potent as beclomethasone and budesonide

Parenteral steroids

Use lowest dose possible for adequate control
Adults: give as single morning dose
Children: use alternate morning single dose (average maintenance dose up to 1 mg/kg/alternate day for prednisolone)

Prednisolone	1 and 5 mg; enteric-coated tablets also available
Deflazacort	6 mg tablets
Triamcinolone acetonide	40 mg/ml: intramuscular injection 1–2 ml

Other controllers

Sodium cromoglycate	Nebulizer solution: 20 mg (2 ml) 3–4 times daily as prophylaxis DPI (Spinhaler): 20 mg 3–4 times daily as prophylaxis MDI (5 mg/puff): 1–2 puffs 4 times daily as prophylaxis
Nedocromil sodium	MDI (2 mg/puff): 2 puffs 2–4 times daily as prophylaxis
Montelukast (an anti-leukotriene)	Tablet (10 mg adult, 5 mg children) once daily in evening as prophylaxis
Slow-release theophylline preparations	Many preparations as prophylaxis Children: build up to about 5 mg/kg twice daily with checks on blood level Adults: build up to about 4 mg/kg twice daily with checks on blood level (NB: These doses are designed to give blood levels in the range of 5–10 mg/l)
Short ('crash') course corticosteroids	Children: Oral prednisolone: start with 2.0 mg/kg/day in divided doses and reduce in steps to zero over 5–10 days provided control is adeqaute. If not, consider higher dose or longer course but courses lasting more than 2–3 weeks are likely to cause side-effects

Adults: Similar to children, but start with prednisolone about 30–40 mg/day and reduce over 7–10 days
Oral steroids may be stopped abruptly rather than tailed down if preferred

Acute (emergency) medications
Bronchodilators
Salbutamol

Nebulized:
Children – 0.15 mg/kg up to 5.0 mg maximum diluted to 2–3 ml with normal saline
Adults – 5.0 mg diluted to 2–3 ml with normal saline
Both – 20 puffs of MDI into large volume spacer

Intravenous:
Children – 0.1–0.2 µg/kg/min
Adults – initially 5 µg/min, then adjust to avoid excessive heart rate response (average 3–20 µg/min)

Terbutaline

Nebulized:
Children – 0.3 mg/kg up to 10 mg maximum, diluted to 2–3 ml with normal saline
Adults – 10 mg diluted to 2–3 ml with normal saline
Both – 20 puffs of MDI into large volume spacer

Intravenous:
Children – 0.02–0.06 µg/kg/min
Adults – 1.5–5.0 µg/min

Ipratropium bromide	Nebulized:
	To be added to β_2-agonist inhalation every 2-4 hours
	Children - 5-7 µg/kg
	Adults - 500 µg (2 ml of 250 µg/ml solution)

Aminophylline

If patient has not been taking theophylline preparations; loading dose of 7 mg/kg up to maximum of 250 mg over 20 min then maintenance of 0.5-1.0 mg/kg/h and measure blood level

If patient has been taking theophylline preparations: no loading dose, only maintenance of 0.5-1.0 mg/kg/h and measure blood level

Corticosteroids

Oral prednisolone
Children - give 2 mg/kg stat, then tail down over 7-10 days
Adults - 60 mg stat, then tail down over 7-10 days

Intravenous hydrocortisone
Children - 4 mg/kg every 6 hours
Adults - 200 mg every 6 hours

Intravenous methylprednisolone
Children - 1-1.5 mg/kg every 6 hours
Adults - 100 mg every 6 hours

Index